To the love of my life. Without your patient love and support, my professional accomplishments would be meaningless.

—Frank

To an amazing partner and the most cherished family, friends, and "greys" with whom I've been blessed. If everyone had people like you to love, the world would be such a better place.

—Zella

Contents

PART I. THEORETICAL AND EMPIRICAL FOUNDATIONS

List of Figures

Preface

The development of the Mindfulness-Acceptance-Commitment (MAC) approach to performance enhancement, and ultimately this text, is a testament to the way in which the science-practice connection in professional psychology is intended to work. That is, practice issues should guide scientific inquiry, which, in turn, should directly inform innovative empirically developed methods capable of being applied in the real world.

Long ago, the first author (Gardner) dutifully utilized traditional performance enhancement techniques and strategies in his work with elite athletes and business professionals. Unfortunately, they really didn't work very well, and the less-than-stellar outcomes produced by these approaches were at first quite daunting and humbling. It was only after many years of discussions with peer-colleagues at conferences and within social-professional circles that it became clear that most professionals utilizing such techniques privately noted a similarly troubling lack of success when using traditional psychological skills training procedures. Of course, we all tried to remember those clients who improved dramatically with the use of our methods, just as the weekend golfer tries to remember the one or two great shots that were surrounded by 115 very poor ones. There had to be something better. We were all searching. As Gardner looks back and celebrates his 20-year anniversary working in professional sports, one can't help but think of all the high performing individuals who deserved to improve in their given domains to the same extent that clinical patients were able to improve following scientifically grounded, empirically supported interventions that truly targeted and remediated their concerns. Yet, nothing really existed to help the performer in truly sustainable ways, and, as such, we watched as sport and performance psychology teetered to survive at the consumer level.

Following hours of listening to Gardner's disgruntled commentary about the state of the sport and performance psychology field, the second author (Moore), who was just entering the professional world of performance psychology, decided to painstakingly and systematically evaluate the empirical support for these traditional methods. Of course, if one were to simply listen to the efficacy statements presented in self-help and professional texts or what professionals presented at national conferences, one would have assumed that these were sound methods for the enhancement of performance. But we knew better, as do many professional in the sport and performance domains. So Moore gathered the data on the efficacy of these procedures with competitive athletes, which was reported in peer-reviewed journals. As described in chapter 2, it became clear that the data matched the experiences and private conversations of professional sport and performance psychologists. The analysis suggested a troubling absence of empirical evidence for the efficacy of the traditional methods of performance enhancement. As such, these results called for us to once again go back to the theory-building stage and, ultimately, to the development of new and innovative psychological interventions for performance enhancement.

Our theory-building process (described in chapter 1) connected the scientific knowledge base on human performance and self-regulation, and more contemporary findings related to metacognitive processes, emotion regulation, and acceptance-based behavioral interventions. This process led to the theory and practical application of the MAC program. The development of MAC from theory to protocol, and from empirical evaluation to practical application, finally led to the development of this text. This has been an exciting professional adventure that we are excited to share. While we have received much positive feedback about the application of this approach, we fervently hope that this text will spur researchers to become involved in further evaluation of the MAC approach, because such inquiry is a fundamental requirement of any true scientific discipline and is certainly how those committed to evidence-based practice operate.

Our expectation is that some professionals committed to traditional psychological skills training methods and techniques will ignore or blindly criticize this new approach. This is fine but will be yet another disappointing acknowledgement of the binary approach to sport and performance psychology that has stunted the growth of the field for decades. Our hope is that students and practitioners alike will consider the material presented in this book with an open yet scientifically skeptical mind. Our intent is to provide the practitioner-scientist with a new way of thinking about the relationship between one's inner experiences and high-level human performance and the ways that we, as professionals, can influence that relationship. With this in mind, this text has been written as a user-friendly practitioner's guide that can serve as a step-by-step intervention manual. We provide all of the theoretical, empirical, and practical tools necessary for using the MAC program with a variety of high-performing clientele. This text represents a milestone in our professional lives, and we hope that this work can contribute to the enhancement of readers' professional performance and the performance of their clients for many years to come. To further enhance the utilization of the MAC program, the exercises and forms in this book are accessible and downloadable via the Springer Publishing Company Web site (www.springerpub.com). When you click on the link you will be asked for a password. The password is macform07.

Acknowledgments

The development of the Mindfulness-Acceptance-Commitment approach to performance enhancement was the result of years of hard work on both of our parts. The stagnation in sport and performance psychology domains, and the fascinating scientific developments within clinical psychology primed us to reconsider, reformulate, and finally construct a new theoretical and practical approach to enhancing human performance. After developing the MAC protocol, we were struck with how many professionals seemed to just "get it" and frequently asked us for more information on how they could integrate this approach into their own practice with high-performing clientele. We found ourselves inspired, and thus embarked on the creation of this book. We genuinely hope that practitioners will embrace this approach to performance enhancement, and will enjoy the same feeling that we get when we see our clients improve in fundamental, substantial, and sustainable ways. From our personal experiences (and the reported experiences of others), there are not many approaches to performance enhancement that seem to have the same effect on performers' lives, either in performance or general life domains. We are so eager for your clients to begin their new lives, and we are therefore pleased that you have embarked on this journey.

Many influential people deserve our thanks and appreciation. We first extend tremendous thanks to our families and friends for their support, sacrifice, and overwhelming love. Second, we also thank our professional families. Frank would like to thank the students, faculty, and administration at La Salle University in Philadelphia, Pennsylvania, especially within the Departments of Psychology and Athletics. Zella's appreciation goes out to her professional family at Manhattan College in New York City, where she is supported by amazing undergraduate students, faculty colleagues, and administration. We endlessly thank the dedicated staff at Springer, especially Sheri W. Sussman and Alana Stein, for their patience, support, encouragement, and commitment to scientific advancement.

Finally, we sincerely thank our professional colleagues worldwide who are interested in new scientific developments and committed to providing their clients with the best possible care. Because of practitioners committed to evidence-based practice, the world is truly a better place.

PART I

Theoretical and Empirical Foundations

CHAPTER 1

Understanding Functional and Dysfunctional Human Performance: The Integrative Model of Human Performance

It can probably be stated that experts rule the world. At the very least, they typically garner high levels of respect, make forward-thinking decisions, have valued opinions, and gain praise for their admirable achievements. Indeed, everyone cannot achieve this honorable status. Just one step below the expert lie numerous talented individuals who act as the expert's support system, carrying out those activities that allow the expert to maintain peak success. But why do so many people plateau just below the expert level, striving to become true experts but only warranting terms such as *talented, great,* a *go-getter,* and *valuable*? Is there really such a difference in the technical skills and abilities of the expert and the *valuable* coworker, teammate, or associate?

As a complex human activity, multiple factors—both internal and external—are intricately tied to understanding, predicting, and enhancing human performance. As such, it is not reasonable to focus on any one activity, mechanism, or variable as being responsible for all the internal and external concerns that enhance or impede human performance. This chapter and the intervention protocol that follows seek to better understand and, in turn, ultimately influence human performance through understanding how internal processes interact with external demands.

Naturally, many factors determine the effectiveness of human performance. The myriad of factors contributing to functional as well as dysfunctional human performance can be summarized as follows:

- **Instrumental competencies:** These include an individual's specific physical/sensorimotor and/or cognitive skills and abilities.
- **Environmental stimuli and performance demands:** These include the work, competitive, interpersonal, situational, and organizational circumstances, issues, and challenges that the performer must face.
- **Dispositional characteristics:** These include intrapersonal (i.e., within-person) characteristics such as coping styles (approach/avoidance), and cognitive-affective schemas, which are the psychological templates by which the performer perceives, interprets, and responds to explicit and implicit performance stimuli and demands.
- **Behavioral self-regulation:** This includes interconnected cognitive, affective, physiological, and behavioral processes that are the foundation of goal-directed behavior within any performance domain.

When these four components are appropriately aligned, what results is an ideal performance state (Hardy, Jones, & Gould, 1996). Several authors have discussed the concept of an ideal performance state using varying terminology. Csikszentmihalyi (1975) described this state, characterized by automatic, effortless attention to task, as "flow," while Gould and Udry (1994), in their description of necessary factors for creating an ideal performance state, used the term "recipe of emotions." Finally, Hanin (1980) used the phrase "zone of optimal functioning" to describe the idiographic arousal state necessary for optimal performance. All of these terms suggest that underlying elite levels of human performance is an optimal biopsychosocial state that promotes and sustains automated, task-focused, goal-directed behavior. In essence, the right combination of cognitive, affective, and physiological conditions allows well-learned skills to occur in a seemingly effortless and automatic manner. This chapter focuses on how this occurs and on what processes promote or interfere with optimal performance.

The model of functional and dysfunctional human performance presented here involves three broad yet interactive phases. When we originally created the model, we called it the Integrative Model of Athletic Performance (IMAP), because it was first designed to highlight the processes by which athletes attain and maintain optimal performance states. The model has since been expanded to aid in the understanding of other high performance domains as well. Thus, we altered the term from IMAP to the Integrative Model of Human Performance (IMHP). Nonetheless, the three interactive phases remain the same. First, the *preperformance phase* involves internal and external demands and processes that promote readiness for competitive or performance-related behavior and, as such, involves factors that are present prior to actual performance. The *performance phase* involves the interaction of cognitive, affective, physiological, and behavioral processes during performance, including skill execution. The *postperformance response phase* involves responses to performance outcomes, and is present following competitive performance.

PREPERFORMANCE PHASE

Regardless of the performance area, performers of all types possess an array of specific skills and personal abilities, and these skills and abilities are likely to differ based on age, competitive/work level, and type of activity. Yet an individual's level of performance is not simply based on whether the individual possesses the right combination of traits, physical capacity, and skill sets. If that were the case, many more people would be considered experts, and the term *expert* would not evoke such respect and admiration. In addition to physical skills and personal abilities, the performer is also impacted by internal dispositional characteristics, environmental stimuli, and performance demands.

Dispositional Characteristics

Dispositional characteristics are the template for the assimilation and accommodation of environmental stimuli. In this regard, the professional literature in both clinical and cognitive psychology suggests that individuals develop an interactive pattern of self and other mental schemas (internal rule systems) as cognitive representations of the self and its relation to the world based on repeated life experiences (Safran & Segal, 1990). These internal representations are implicit cognitive structures that influence the performer's allocation of attention to stimuli that are perceived as either physically or psychologically dangerous. Schemas serve as a basis for understanding the world, controlling emotional responses, and maintaining interpersonal relatedness. In essence, schemas serve as personal radar from which an individual scans for possible (psychological) threat, which results in learned patterns of cognitive, affective, and behavioral responses to the world.

Of course, all individuals develop some verbal/linguistic representations based on their personal learning histories. The development of such rule systems and ways of viewing the world greatly helps people organize information and make sense of new material and experiences. In this regard, schemas can be quite necessary and adaptive. On the other hand, some individuals develop more strongly held and problematic schematic representations due to more challenging or chronic learning histories. For such persons, behavior will frequently be guided more by these relatively inflexible verbal networks than by environmental realities and the contingencies in their world. As a result, and again based largely on the individual's previous learning experiences, attentional biases related to these schemas develop as the individual misclassifies innocuous stimuli in the environment (Teachman & Woody, 2004). This leads such individuals to act in ways that are inconsistent with the demands of their environment, and such persons may even act against their chosen values and goals. Simply put, in these circumstances, behavior is directed more by the individual's internal processes (cognitions, affect, and physiological sensations) than by environmental needs and consequences. For instance, the individual may choose behaviors aimed at reducing how bad one feels, rather than choosing to engage in more functional behaviors that promote the individual's overall best interest.

Rigid behavioral patterns associated with these internal processes are often referred to as *rule-governed behaviors*. In such circumstances, behavior is governed by rigid internal rules rather than by the needs and necessities of the environment. Self-defeating response patterns may result, as the psychological self-protective function (i.e., avoidance of emotional discomfort) of these schemas often occurs at the expense of more functional behavior, such as acting in the service of one's goals and values. As a more complex example, consider an individual who would like to develop intimate relationships with others but, because of a difficult personal history, has developed a rule system suggesting that relationships are likely to result in pain. This individual is likely to manifest a behavioral pattern of interpersonal avoidance and thus not easily achieve the valued goal of being in a rewarding relationship.

What does this have to do with expert performers or those seeking to attain consistent optimal performance levels? In the context of human performance, the personal meaning and importance the individual places on his or her own performance help form an organizing system by which he or she evaluates, interprets, and responds to the competitive world; and, clearly, how one perceives the environment and the behavioral choices made in response to such perceptions and interpretations significantly contribute to one's success. Of additional importance, if this personal organizing system is combined with a genetic/biological predisposition to experience emotion in a more or less intense manner (often termed *negative affect syndrome* or *neuroticism* by theorists (Barlow, Allen, & Choate,

2004), the result may be an even greater tendency to interpret threat and danger, and may subsequently lead to increased behavioral restriction and distance from perceived (or misperceived) threat.

Environmental Stimuli

Dispositional characteristics make up the essence of the individual and can therefore be viewed as setting the stage for how an individual interprets and responds to the external demands and environmental stimuli of one's competitive situation. We define environmental stimuli as those external factors that the performer confronts both in and out of competition. Personal and professional relationships, organizational/corporate realities and demands, physical and psychological aspects of training and competition (travel, time commitments, etc.), financial pressures, career stage, and physical strain and injury all have stimulus properties that a performer may respond to based on personal learning histories. These are but some of the factors that the high-level performer must successfully confront in order to consistently function at optimal levels.

Performance Demands

In addition to the vast array of environmental challenges and stressors that performers must face, successful individuals are also typically pressured to meet the performance demands and standards set by themselves and others. We define performance demands as the specific cues and general requirements necessary to perform under conditions in which the individual is challenged to achieve *at* or *above* an established standard. While established performance standards vary depending on level and domain (i.e., recreational, collegiate, Olympic, or professional athletes; type of business and type of position held), all levels within each performance domain explicitly and implicitly establish a number of required performance standards.

Why is understanding all of this so important? The interaction of performance-specific skills, dispositional characteristics, environmental stimuli, and performance demands are the precursors for active engagement in actual performance, and this interaction is the context for optimal behavior self-regulation *during* performance endeavors. It is in this context that one's early learning histories, the adaptive and maladaptive verbal rules (schemas) developing from these histories, and the behavioral patterns that follow from these rules can result in either functional performance based on an effective self-regulatory process or dysfunctional performance through the disruption of the self-regulatory process.

PERFORMANCE PHASE

With dispositional characteristics (developed from one's learning history), environmental stimuli, and performance demands in place, the individual performer will experience some degree of physiological arousal and cognitive activity related to his or her performance (and performance evaluation) when confronted with a performance situation. Optimally, individuals will metacognitively (automatically) attend to relevant aspects of their own behavior and systematically utilize reference points to evaluate and adjust their behavior to meet established standards. This process is often referred to as *discrepancy adjustment* (Carver & Scheier, 1988; Wells, 2000). This process of discrepancy adjustment is somewhat analogous to the cruise control mechanism in a motor vehicle. The vehicle notes changes in road conditions and adjusts the speed accordingly to maintain a predetermined desired speed. From a human performance perspective, an individual will note personal cues and cues in the environment and make performance adjustments to attain or maintain a predetermined performance standard.

Yet to engage in discrepancy adjustment during a performance-related task, the individual must self-monitor (attend to) his or her own behavior to determine how it conforms to these preset standards. In all areas of human performance—whether performing surgery, tackling an opponent, or performing in a recital—slight adjustments to one's behavior will occur even if the individual is not fully aware of the adjustment. Similar to the cruise control example, these relevant behaviors will be slightly adjusted in a seemingly automated, metacognitive manner, with the intent to meet preset performance standards (Carver & Scheier, 1988; Sbrocco & Barlow, 1996). Failure to correctly read the demands of the performance situation and appropriately evaluate one's current level of performance will result in failure to make necessary personal adjustments and maintain an effective performance state. Thus, the metacognitive process of self-monitoring, self-evaluation, and corrective action is central to effective behavioral self-regulation and, ultimately, task execution. Although this process may sound daunting, it typically occurs naturally and operates smoothly and automatically for most individuals, thereby leading to generally stable functional performance.

However, for many individuals, performance schemas and environmental disruptions confound this process by creating unreasonable standards or altering existing skill sets. For example, the perfectionist performer with unrelenting performance standards will compare her real or perceived performance with unrealistic and possibly unattainable standards and is thus unable to engage in adaptive discrepancy adjustment. If the presence of rigid preexisting schemas is added to the situation, the performer is unlikely to be amenable to a logical analysis of her exaggerated standards. Similarly, a recently injured athlete whose skill level has temporarily been altered may be unable to make necessary corrective adjustments and may respond with a dysfunctional spiral. In each of these examples, as with all self-regulatory disruption (Sbrocco & Barlow, 1996), there is a deleterious shift from effective behavioral self-regulation based on subtle metacognitive and automatic processes, to a greater utilization of the controlled, effortful verbal-linguistic cognitive processes that often interrupt effective performance. In essence, when the process is automatic, the individual is able to remain essentially task-focused, and when the process becomes overly cognitive, the result is excessive self-focused attention.

Of particular importance is the degree to which the performer shifts from task-focused attention to self-focused attention. Of course, to engage in the naturally occurring self-adjustment process noted above, one *must* focus on the self to some degree. However, the performer exhibiting functional performance experiences a nonjudging, metacognitive mindful absorption in the task, whereas an individual experiencing dysfunctional performance typically focuses on inflexible rule systems (i.e., thoughts about what he or she can or cannot do, should or should not do, etc.), perceived deficits, self-doubts, efforts to control thoughts and emotions, and ramifications of possible failure. During these periods, less attention is placed on the environment (task-focused attention), and attention is placed instead on internal processes such as thoughts and emotions. The concept of *metacognition* used here is congruent with the definition of what has been referred to as *mindfulness*. Mindfulness, a core feature of this text, has been defined as "paying attention in a particular way: on purpose, in the present moment, and non-judgmentally" (Kabat-Zinn, 1994, p. 4). The concept of mindful (present-moment, nonjudging) task absorption as a foundation of functional performance is an extension of similar descriptions of flow or peak experiences as described by Csikszentmihalyi (1990) and our previous work (Gardner & Moore, 2004a).

The accumulated empirical evidence has led to similar findings in studies across many forms of human performance (Barlow, 2002). For example, research in academic test performance suggests that most individuals experience similar physiological arousal during an academic test. However, when equating for academic preparation, those with self-doubts and an attentional focus on task-irrelevant cues during the exam perform most poorly (Rich & Woolever, 1988). This finding is similar to past research in athletic performance that suggested that athletes who interpret somatic arousal as facilitative maintain task-relevant focus and perform adequately, while those who interpret arousal as debilitative focus more on internal processes, which subsequently interfere with competitive performance (Jones, Hanton, & Swain, 1994; Jones, Swain, & Hardy, 1993; Swain & Jones, 1996). The literature on human sexual performance has described similar findings. Individuals who engage in functional sexual performance focus on task-relevant erotic cues, while those experiencing sexual dysfunction focus on task-irrelevant cues such as self-doubts, sexual inadequacies, and exaggerated self-implications regarding performance failures (Jones, Bruce, & Barlow, 1986).

As can be seen in numerous areas of human performance, performers enter into situations—even situations requiring elite activity—with markedly different expectations about their performance, and these expectations typically become the driving force for their performance-relevant behavioral responses (Barlow, 1986; Vealey, 1986). Due to a combination of dispositional characteristics and personal performance histories, functional performers typically expect positive performance outcomes, and dysfunctional performers typically expect negative performance outcomes. Over time, these beliefs become strongly held and difficult to change. In addition, these belief sets can become self-fulfilling because they affect how the performer interprets challenge or threat in performance situations (Sbrocco & Barlow, 1996). For example, in studies comparing sexually dysfunctional and functional individuals, sexually functional participants who were told that they were ingesting a pill (placebo) that would negatively affect sexual arousal responded to this experimental condition as a challenge and demonstrated *greater* sexual arousal. Conversely, sexually dysfunctional individuals interpreted this same condition as a threat and responded with significantly *lower* levels of sexual arousal (Cranston-Cuebas, Barlow, Mitchell, & Athanasiou, 1993). In a study yielding a similar result, sexually functional individuals demonstrated no increase in arousal when presented with a "performance enhancement" pill (which was a placebo) because they believed their performance did not need enhancement and had little expectation that the pill would enhance their performance. Conversely, sexually dysfunctional individuals responded with greater arousal, because they expected enhanced sexual performance from use of the pill (Cranston-Cuebas & Barlow, 1995).

In each of these studies, outcome expectancies mediated performance demands and impacted performance outcomes by leading to different performance behaviors among participants. These results are consistent with the findings of Gould, Weiss, and Weinberg (1981), who found that confidence was the most stable and consistent factor differentiating highly successful from less successful athletes. Performers who believe that their skills and abilities match performance demands are likely to perform better, and performers who question their skills and experience and are overly concerned with outcome are likely to perform more poorly.

POSTPERFORMANCE RESPONSE PHASE

The postperformance response phase typically follows one of three paths. The performer (1) sustains involvement in his or her competitive performance; (2) reengages as required following a brief dysfunctional period; or (3) disengages from the activity covertly (mental disengagement through worry or distraction) or overtly (physical disengagement by feigning illness, skipping practice, or full termination).

When human performance follows a functional trajectory, the performer's ongoing and future performance behavior remains committed, approach-oriented, and directly linked to personal values. That is, the performer tolerates short-term discomfort related to any given poor performance and continues to approach performance cues and demands with committed preparation, training, and practice. Approach behavior may include additional practice or preparation time, additional work with coaches and managers on technical or tactical development, and additional conditioning and learning. With functional performers, motivation remains strong (because goal-directed behavior is reinforced at a relatively high rate), and positive outcome expectations evolve and strengthen. Appropriate focus on performance cues intensifies, which further promotes ongoing skill development. Positive performance outcomes then reinforce the earlier components of the self-regulatory process (such as appropriate discrepancy adjustment) and increase the likelihood of future successful behavior.

Of course, many people would like to think that elite performers have reached that level because they have never experienced adversity, have never had to struggle to learn a skill, or have been handed their elite status. The fact is that, whether performing at elite or subelite levels, *all* performers experience adversity. Yet, even when faced with performance adversity, the individual with a positive learning history of performance who does not hold extreme maladaptive performance schemas, who has maintained reasonably positive outcome expectations, and who is generally experientially accepting is not likely to overinterpret the personal meaning or future ramifications of any specific negative performance or become unwilling to experience short-term discomfort in the pursuit of his or her goals and values. This performer thus reengages in the performance task as the cues and demands of the competitive situation dictate, even when experiencing less-than-optimal performance. In this situation, negative performance is typically viewed as an isolated episode and does not interfere with adaptive coping (approach) behaviors. This type of individual effectively problem solves and focuses on skill development or on enhancing technical and tactical aspects of performance with a minimum of negative affect.

Some performers, however, respond much differently to negative performances, and a chronic or debilitating performance trajectory may occur. In some performers, discrepancy adjustment difficulties can negatively affect performance, but the performers quickly recover because of adaptive dispositional characteristics; a high trait level of experiential acceptance (i.e., willingness to experience internal events); and/or positive outcome expectancies that isolate the temporary dysfunction as situational, nonthreatening, and tolerable. However, for other performers, changing external circumstances such as a higher level of competition or a new, possibly less supportive organization can trigger preexisting performance schemas, problematic levels of experiential avoidance (i.e., avoidance of the experience of negative internal processes such as thoughts, feelings, and sensations), and skill disruption. Such individuals often respond with persistent performance dysfunction that may be temporary (a slump) or chronic and pervasive.

A study by Klinger, Barta, and Glas (1981) provides some support for this conceptualization of functional and dysfunctional performance. Utilizing thought sampling with college basketball players, their study suggested that, in response to decrements in team performance or a strong challenge from the opposing team, athletes often shift attention from game-related contextual (external) cues and demands to excessive self-focus on both behavior and internal experiences. It can be hypothesized that athletes who hold generally positive outcome expectancies maintain a committed, approach-oriented coping style when faced with performance adversity; continue to engage in the athletic task; and eventually find their way back to functional performance through effective problem solving or coaching. This approach-based coping strategy is likely to result only in brief, time-limited performance decrements.

Chronic performance dysfunction, however, is much more likely to be associated with an avoidant coping style. This style may be overlearned from childhood or develop gradually in response to the repeated failure of more adaptive efforts toward successful performance reengagement. These may be true negative experiences in which poor outcomes occurred, or they may be negative experiences in which premature cessation or termination of performance occurred due to an unwillingness to experience the increase in negative thoughts, emotions, or physiological sensations associated with performance situations. Consistent with social-cognitive models of motivation and goal seeking behavior (Carver & Scheier, 1988), individuals typically remain task-engaged as long as they reasonably believe that positive outcomes are likely, and they disengage when negative outcomes (broadly defined) are consistently anticipated. From this perspective, the performer experiencing chronic or persistent performance dysfunction is likely to respond with either behavioral or cognitive avoidance.

Behavioral Avoidance

To fully understand behavioral avoidance, we must understand the function of this strategy. Inherent in our conceptualization of performance dysfunction and consistent with recent research on behavior disorders (Hayes, Wilson, Gifford, Follette, & Strosahl, 1996) is the idea that experiential avoidance functions to provide the individual experiencing heightened negative affect a means of short-term emotion regulation. Although experiential avoidance does not fulfill long-term goals and values, it does immediately reduce negative emotion and, as such, is strongly (negatively) reinforced. The individual often learns and generalizes this reinforced pattern across numerous life situations, but the pattern can also develop specifically in the competitive performance context. Behavioral avoidance strategies can be overt in the form of complete disengagement from the performance context (such as quitting a job or retiring from sport) or can be covert and less obvious (such as finding reasons to not come to work). For example, an individual is required to have a quarterly accounts meeting with his manager, yet each time the meeting approaches, he finds a reason to postpone the meeting due to his increasing anxiety. While the strategy does nothing to improve his sales performance or enhance his relationship with his manager, it does serve the immediate function of reducing the anxiety and is thus negatively reinforced.

When performance dysfunction becomes more long-term and chronic, however, task disengagement may become more obvious and complete. Repeated failure to perform at expected standards can extinguish approach behaviors and negatively reinforces avoidant behaviors such as complete withdrawal from the activity in question. As Smith (1986) suggested, the balance between reinforcement and the aversive consequences of continued participation in a given activity becomes such that dissatisfaction and negative affect predominate. The cost-benefit analysis of continued participation in the given activity often leads to complete disengagement from active participation. This phenomenon has been termed *burnout* (Hardy et al., 1996; Smith, 1986).

Cognitive Avoidance

Cognitive avoidance can take the form of processes such as worry and rumination, which are naturally occurring processes that, at nonpathological levels, serve an important problem-solving function. At nonpathological levels, they adaptively prepare individuals to confront challenge or threat.

Yet when excessive, these cognitive processes are linked to anxiety and deleterious performance ramifications. In this regard, Borkovec (1994) presented a theoretical formulation describing the process and function of both extreme (clinical) and nonpathological worry. In his formulation, worry is a covert verbal-linguistic (also known as verbal-semantic) activity that allows individuals to *avoid* the complete experience of negative affect or affect-provoking stimuli. Driven by initial signs of arousal, the verbal-linguistic process of worry occupies one's attentional focus and effectively suppresses the full experience of anxiety (Barlow, 2002) or other affective responses such as sadness, guilt, or anger (Gardner & Moore, in press). Importantly, Borkovec also noted that, unlike anxiety (which is associated with increased physiological arousal), worry has a distinctive physiological process of sympathetic arousal *restriction,* which has been viewed as evidence of the inability of individuals engaged in worry to fully experience the physiological components of anxiety. Worry essentially inhibits the affective-physiological arousal components of anxiety and is thus negatively reinforced for the individual. Therefore, while at nonpathological levels cognitive processes such as worry and rumination are coping strategies that can aid in problem solving, at more pathological levels they are avoidance strategies that subsequently disengage the performer from necessary task-focused attention and lead to ineffective behavioral choices.

Some of the studies supporting Borkovec's formulation are particularly relevant to performance psychology. Studies of both pathological and nonpathological worry suggest that individuals who worry report more thoughts than images during the worry process (Borkovec, 1994; Borkovec & Inz, 1990; Freeston, Dugas, & Ladouceur, 1996). In a study in which participants were instructed to worry while engaging in tasks that were primarily either verbal or visuospatial, worry interfered with only the verbal tasks, thus demonstrating its verbal-linguistic nature (Rapee, 1993). Bergman and Craske (1994) found that individuals preparing for public speaking shifted from visualizing a neutral scene to verbal-linguistic activity as they began to worry about the imminent task. In another study, individuals engaged in a worry task demonstrated increased frontal cortical activation in the left hemisphere, thus indicating increased verbal-linguistic activation (Carter, Johnson, & Borkovec, 1986). This finding is particularly important in the context of an additional study by Crews and Landers (1993), which found that highly skilled golfers engaging in a competitive putting task demonstrated a significant increase in left hemispheric alpha activity indicative of reduced verbal-linguistic processes. To clarify this important finding, the golfers who performed better experienced less cognitive activity (thought less) than those who performed more poorly. This study provides some evidence for an inverse relationship between internal verbal processes and athletic performance. Similar results have been found in additional studies of elite marksmen and archers (Hatfield, Landers, & Ray, 1984; Janelle, Hillman, Apparies, et al., 2000; Janelle, Hillman, & Hatfield, 2000; Salazar, Landers, Petruzzello, & Han, 1990). From this empirical base, it seems reasonable to conclude that worry—a process associated with *increased* cognitive activity—may particularly impede optimal athletic performance, because optimal performance seems to require *reduced* cognitive activity (i.e., a quiet mind).

Borkovec's (1994) empirically informed conceptualization of worry may also explain the conflicting and inconsistent findings in the sport and performance psychology literature examining the relationship between competitive anxiety and athletic performance (McNally, 2002). The multidimensional theory of competitive trait anxiety (Martens, Burton, Vealey, Bump, & Smith, 1990) and the cusp-catastrophe model of the anxiety-performance relationship both utilize the concept of cognitive anxiety, defining it as fear of failure and negative expectations about performance (Hardy et al., 1996). Woodman and Hardy (2001) referred to cognitive anxiety and worry as synonymous terms. At present, despite the empirical data suggesting otherwise, the sport psychology literature does not clearly distinguish worry and anxiety. It is important to note that, while worry is a fundamental component of all types of anxiety (Barlow, 2002), recent evidence confirms that worry is a functional process that is more than just a symptom of anxiety. The inconsistencies in the sport science research relating to the relative impact of cognitive or somatic anxiety on competitive performance (McNally, 2002) may be explained by the fact that the most frequently used theoretical models describing the relationship between anxiety and performance do not consider and incorporate the construct of worry and its effects on performance independently of its contribution to the negative affective state of anxiety. In fact, clinical scientists have suggested that worry and anxiety are partially independent constructs (Craske, 1999; Davey, Hampton, Farrell, & Davidson, 1992).

One may wonder why noting the distinction between worry and anxiety is so important for a performance psychology text. Our goal is for the protocol presented in this text to allow the performer to overcome his or her obstacles and reach the highest level of performance attainable based on personal skills and abilities. With that said, while mild worry serves an adaptive function by aiding in the process of planning for possible negative events and reducing the seemingly unpredictable and uncontrollable nature of these events, we believe that maladaptive, covert expressions of experiential avoidance (such as worry) hinder the performer's ability to reach valued long-term goals and only serve to immediately reduce discomfort. But everyone experiences discomfort—it is *natural*—and, while worry may successfully remove immediate discomfort in the short term, it does not help develop the skills necessary for optimal performance. Particularly problematic, worry also can become highly automated and resistant to change. The performer utilizing worry as a covert avoidance strategy in response to performance decrements tends to sustain his or her performance difficulties by disrupting the automated execution of skills as worry loops back and negatively influences self-regulation in the preperformance, performance, or postperformance response phases. In the latter phase, the overuse of task-avoidant worry is likely to interfere with both effective problem solving (leading to decreased practice, poor training intensity, and self-care considerations) and skill modification and development in response to short-term performance difficulties.

INTRODUCTION TO THE ACCEPTANCE-BASED APPROACH

Traditional models of human performance have often focused on negative emotions and distorted or dysfunctional content of one's thoughts (negative thoughts about performance) as central to understanding performance difficulties. Yet more recently, theorists, researchers, and practitioners have considered a more contemporary acceptance-based approach to understanding such psychological phenomena (Gardner & Moore, 2004a; Hayes, Strosahl, & Wilson, 1999; Orsillo & Roemer, 2005). Contrary to traditional models, we use an acceptance-based approach to suggest that, during the performance phase—which is the point of the self-regulatory process in which physiological arousal, cognitions relating to performance and performance evaluation, emotional reactivity, and self-awareness of these changes (self-focused attention) increase—it is the degree of *experiential acceptance* displayed by the performer that is critical to ultimate performance outcomes. In other words, performance outcomes depend on the degree to which the performer accepts his or her own internal experiences as normal and naturally occurring; is willing to persist on task despite these experiences; and maintains attentional focus on the environmental task at hand rather than on his or her internal thoughts, feelings, and physical sensations. Along these lines, it is not the presence or absence of negative thoughts, physiological arousal, or emotions such as anxiety or anger that predicts performance outcomes; rather, it is the degree to which the individual performer can accept these experiences and remain attentionally and behaviorally engaged in the performance task. When experiential acceptance occurs, attentional focus remains on the necessary aspects of the performance environment, and the performer will simply notice the cognitive, affective, and physiological arousal without the need to control, escape, or avoid it. As such, the impact of these internal states on performance will be minimal. Conversely, in the context of low experiential acceptance, which is termed *experiential avoidance* (Hayes et al., 1999), the performer is likely to engage in a variety of control strategies designed to alter the content and intensity of these internal experiences and the rate at which they occur. Common control strategies include self-talk, thought suppression, distraction, and termination of performance effort. On occasion, these control strategies may briefly succeed by reducing one's immediate discomfort, but they are most often bound to fail and frequently lead to further increases in arousal. This is because a vicious cycle begins in which increased arousal, increased self-focused attention, and increased efforts at experiential control result in more behavioral disruption as the performer becomes preoccupied with reducing his or her unpleasant thoughts, feelings, and/or physiological sensations. In addition, the individual will also begin to scan the self for subtle signs of personal discomfort and negative thoughts, thereby reducing the amount of attention the individual can place on necessary performance tasks. These disruptions often begin by leading to mildly impaired competitive performance and, for some individuals, can eventually result in complete avoidance of performance situations.

How does the acceptance-based model fit with Hanin's (1980) individual zones of optimal performance model (IZOP), which suggests that optimal performance is directly related to individually determined optimal levels of emotion? The acceptance-based model of human performance presented herein can be seen as consistent with the IZOP model in the following way. From an acceptance-based theoretical perspective, Hanin's findings in support of the IZOP model may reflect the varying degrees of experiential acceptance and avoidance found across individuals. In this context, variations in performance may not be due to the absolute level of affect experienced, but rather to the degree to which an individual can tolerate (i.e., accept) the experience of that emotion. While this explanation is clearly an open empirical question, we suggest that experiential acceptance/avoidance may mediate the relationship between emotion and performance in the IZOP model.

Using the scientific literature on human performance, we summarize that the following sequence is directly involved in functional performance: (1) Functional performance involves a metacognitive (automated) process of self-monitoring, self-evaluation, and corrective action as needed and does not involve heightened cognitive activity to control or modify internal experiences. (2) The functional processes of effective discrepancy adjustment and experiential acceptance feed into the performer's positive performance expectations (self-efficacy), and the performer interprets performance demands as challenging. (3) This results in further mindful task focus, appropriate levels of arousal and affect, automated motor skills, and, ultimately, in functional performance. Conversely, ineffective discrepancy adjustment leads to interpretations of performance cues and demands as threatening, and, with low levels of experiential acceptance, the individual may engage in a task-irrelevant focus and set of behaviors, become self-judging, scan the environment for signs of threat, and engage in self-focused attention. This set of responses is often associated with heightened negative affect, heightened arousal, reduced concentration, disruption of automated motor skills, and, ultimately, dysfunctional performance. Disruptions in self-regulated performance may occur in acute episodes or become a habitual (overlearned) pattern resulting in chronic performance dysfunction. Preexisting performance schemas and related psychological processes may strongly influence whether episodes of dysfunctional performance become chronic or remain situational.

IMPLICATIONS

Numerous authors have noted the extreme pressures and environmental demands that elite performers must confront (Andersen, 2002; Baillie & Ogilvie, 2002). It has been suggested that competitive performance demands are more likely to tax an individual's personal and social resources than many other human endeavors. This is, of course, in addition to the normative demands of being a spouse, parent, child, friend, coworker, employee, or teammate and dealing with financial, educational, occupational, and living concerns. It is, therefore, crucial to consider all psychological issues, behavioral styles, and life stressors that covertly and overtly impair or delay one's functioning. A truly comprehensive practice model of performance psychology will do no less. Unfortunately, perusal of the theoretical and empirical literature related to traditional performance enhancement strategies suggests that psychological responses to transitional or developmental issues and dispositional psychological characteristics are a relatively unnecessary focus of intervention for enhancing performance (Rotella, 1990). In our opinion, this view is partially responsible for both the stunted growth of performance psychology and the development of ineffective practice models. In addition, the vast majority of the intervention strategies in performance psychology have not been developed to target the specific psychological *processes* involved in human performance and are typically focused on modifying *outcomes* without targeting the real issues. Psychological skills training procedures, the predominant intervention methodologies in applied sport and performance psychology, tend to focus on performance outcomes with little clear connection to the empirically based processes involved in human performance. In contrast, the model of functional and dysfunctional performance described in this chapter clearly suggests that efforts to enhance human performance must be a comprehensive enterprise targeting those specific *processes* in need of development or remediation.

Unlike other performance models—especially those within the sport psychology domain—it is not reasonable to artificially separate performance demands, skills, dispositional variables, and self-regulatory skills in understanding human performance. The arbitrary separation of these constructs would only be possible if, during performance situations, performers could abandon their internal states, rid themselves of dispositional factors (such as personality), set aside life demands, and equalize talent and skill among other performers. Yet performers are not simply "performers," and like all humans, they take physical skills, dispositional variables, and self-regulatory processes with them as they engage in all of life's demands. And, like all humans, these intrapersonal and interpersonal factors can either enhance or impede their chosen endeavors. To utilize a model of human performance that does not fully respect and consider these processes would be futile and ineffectual. In fact, the suggestion that performance can be enhanced apart from this comprehensive understanding contradicts both theoretical and empirical data relating to human performance. Within the Integrative Model of Human Performance, addressing the skill, dispositional, environmental, and self-regulatory issues confronting the performer is both central and critical to promoting the client's performance *and* well-being. At its most fundamental level, the IMHP suggests a completely integrated relationship between these factors and human performance and has clear and logical intervention implications.

Alternative acceptance-based behavioral interventions such as mindfulness and metacognitive procedures for enhancing task-focused attention; acceptance and commitment procedures for behavioral activation and valued goal attainment; and interventions focusing on exposure and response prevention for anxiety and anger-related concerns are indicated for many individuals presenting with performance concerns or desiring an extra advantage or "edge." These interventions, often viewed as "therapeutic," are certainly, in and of themselves, performance-enhancement interventions. We think that the term *performance enhancement* is more appropriate as a statement of *outcome* rather than a definition of a particular intervention technique. Others have also suggested the performance effects of more therapeutic interventions; Giges (2000) stated that the removal of psychological barriers is "an effective method in helping athletes improve their performance" (p. 18).

CONCLUSION

The Integrative Model of Human Performance has been developed by carefully integrating the current literature in clinical and sport science to provide a theoretical understanding of the internal and external components of functional and dysfunctional human performance. This theoretical framework ultimately drives the assessment and intervention processes, which are intended to promote the psychosocial well-being and competitive performance of high-level performers. Using the IMHP as a guide to understanding the processes involved in functional and dysfunctional human performance, the professional can set out to consider the specific processes in need of targeting in the course of performance-enhancement efforts. This will lead to an intervention focus not on outcomes per se, but rather on the processes that underlie optimal performance. This allows for clearer case conceptualization and more rationally determined intervention foci.

This discussion has explained how interpersonal, intrapersonal, environmental, and self-regulatory processes affect both the performance and psychosocial functioning of individual performers. Certainly, performers do not function solely in the competitive domain, but function in many life domains that also require attention and occasional assistance. With the IMHP in mind, chapter 2 begins by discussing the empirical efficacy of traditional skills-based approaches to performance enhancement and introduces the Mindfulness-Acceptance-Commitment approach to performance enhancement, which will be the primary focus for the remainder of the text.

CHAPTER 2

From Change to Acceptance: The Mindfulness-Acceptance-Commitment Approach to Performance Enhancement

It is likely that readers of this text have already utilized performance enhancement efforts to maximize their clients' performance in a variety of occupational, recreational, and general life domains. Some readers may wonder why we have taken a different approach than traditional theoretical models of performance and what this new intervention approach is all about.

For the past three decades, the predominant psychological approach to the enhancement of performance has been techniques and strategies evolving out of the skills-training wing of the cognitive behavioral tradition (Meichenbaum, 1977). These approaches have emphasized the development of self-control of internal states such as thoughts, emotions, and physical sensations and have been commonly referred to as psychological skills training (PST) procedures (Whelan, Mahoney, & Meyers, 1991). From this theoretical perspective, performers develop and utilize mental skills as a means of controlling internal processes with the hope of creating the ideal performance state.

The self-regulatory PST procedures most often discussed are goal-setting, imagery/mental rehearsal, arousal control, self-talk modification, precompetitive routines, and some combination of the above. *Goal-setting* refers to procedures that promote the establishment of short-, medium-, and long-range goals that focus on outcomes, individual performance, or processes. It has been suggested that goal-setting procedures motivate individuals to become more productive and effective (Locke & Latham, 1990). *Imagery* has been defined as procedures that encourage "using all the senses to re-create an experience in the mind" (Vealey & Garner-Holman, 1998, p. 248). Imagery is often used to prepare a performer to correctly execute a skill. *Arousal control* methods (also called arousal regulation) are used to promote personal control over physiological arousal levels, which traditional self-regulation theory suggests must be at an optimal level for effective performance (Hardy et al., 1996). Arousal control methods include variants of relaxation techniques intended to reduce arousal and methods intended to "psych up" or energize individuals when it is deemed that their arousal is too low to successfully engage in performance tasks. *Self-talk* modification procedures are based on models of performance that suggest a simple, linear relationship between thoughts, feelings, and performance. Techniques such as cognitive restructuring and construction and learning of self-affirmations (positive self-talk) are used to enhance performance by controlling thought content and emotional states (Hardy et al., 1996). Finally, *precompetitive routines* are analogous to stimulus control procedures frequently used in behavioral psychology; these methods encourage a consistent sequence of behaviors (both verbal behaviors/thoughts and motor behaviors/actions) preceding performance situations. These procedures are believed to enhance attention through minimizing the presence of distracting stimuli and thereby are believed to promote optimal levels of performance (Hardy et al., 1996).

It has been theorized that the use of these procedures leads to enhanced motivation, confidence, attention, emotional control, and self-awareness—all of which are theorized to, in some way, make it more likely that an individual will better regulate his or her behavior, which in turn creates a necessary condition for optimal performance. The question for the practitioner seeking to engage in an evidence-based practice of his or her discipline is the following: Despite years of use and strong statements about their utility from recognized and well-respected professionals, have these procedures truly demonstrated empirical (i.e., scientific) support for use as a means of enhancing performance?

THE EFFICACY OF TRADITIONAL PST PROCEDURES

The efficacy of psychological skills training techniques and procedures for performance enhancement has been most carefully evaluated within the context of athletic performance enhancement. Historically, numerous authors have supported the use of PST procedures for enhancing athletic performance while commenting on the inconsistent and generally inconclusive empirical support for these procedures (Burton, Naylor, & Holliday, 2001; Gould, Damarjian, & Greenleaf, 2002; Meyers, Whelan, & Murphy, 1996; Weinberg, 2002; Williams & Leffingwell, 2002; Zaichkowsy & Baltzell, 2001). In fact, inconsistent and cautious reviews have been published time and time again. Yet these same reviews frequently conclude by stating that, despite such cautions and inconclusive evidence of efficacy among empirical studies, there is still unequivocal support for the use of PST procedures to enhance performance. We found this to be a baffling and troubling pattern and set out to conduct our own careful and extensive qualitative review of the PST literature. Findings, to be discussed below, suggest that serious questions exist regarding the efficacy of traditional psychological skills training procedures for the enhancement of human performance.

In response to the inconsistencies in the scientific literature regarding the efficacy of the most common interventions utilized for performance enhancement, Moore (second author of this text) conducted a structured qualitative review of the empirical evidence for the use of psychological skills training procedures to enhance competitive athletic performance (originally conducted in 2003 and updated in 2005; Gardner & Moore, 2006; Moore, 2003b). This study utilized the criteria for the determination of empirical support of psychological procedures established by the American Psychological Association's Division 12 (Society for Clinical Psychology) Task Force for the Promotion and Dissemination of Psychological Procedures (Chambless & Hollon, 1998). Using this carefully constructed (and anti-meta-analysis) criteria adopted by numerous other disciplines in professional psychology (Kendall & Chambless, 1998; Spirito, 1999), the purpose of this structured investigation was to effectively evaluate the current empirical support for these common procedures to provide clear direction for researchers and to clarify for practitioners the precise level of scientific empirical support so that they could make more informed intervention decisions that would best meet the needs of their clientele.

The results of this large-scale, structured, qualitative review of the empirical literature on the use of goal-setting, imagery, self-talk, arousal regulation, and multicomponent (i.e., combined procedure) psychological skills training interventions for the enhancement of competitive athletic performance are not encouraging. In fact, despite positive claims from well-respected figures and supportive anecdotal evidence and case study reports, these interventions demonstrate vastly insufficient evidence for their efficacy.

A summary of the findings is provided below; for a comprehensive review, refer to Gardner and Moore (2006, pp. 63–96).

Goal-Setting

Despite the near universal belief that goal-setting procedures are gold-standard techniques for the enhancement of performance, only six empirical studies were found that evaluated the impact of goal-setting on competitive athletic performance (clearly, competitive performers are the target audience, as analogue populations are not sufficient to determine intervention efficacy). Of these six studies, only two met necessary criteria for adequacy of research design (as established by the Division 12 Task Force). Neither of these two studies found any significant performance-enhancing effects for goal-setting procedures. While Locke and Latham (1990)—the major developers and proponents of goal-setting theory and procedures—stated that there is ample evidence to support the use of goal-setting in industrial and organizational settings, these claims await careful independent review. Although not inconsistent with previous cautions suggesting that the performance-enhancing effects of goal-setting have not been established (Dishman, 1983; Meyers et al., 1996; Smith, 1989; Strean & Roberts, 1992), the results of Moore's study are in stark contrast with popular beliefs and current practices in sport and performance psychology, where goal-setting is presented and taught as though it is a highly effective technique that will enhance performance.

Imagery

Moore found similar findings with respect to imagery, another technique considered to be a best-practices procedure within sport psychology. Only seven studies evaluated the use of imagery with competitive performers, and, of those, six met basic research design criteria. Of those six, none demonstrated performance-enhancing effects of imagery. Again, these results, while consistent with numerous cautions, contrast with the way imagery is presented and valued as a performance enhancement tool.

Self-Talk Modification

Similar results were found for self-talk modification procedures. Seven studies using self-talk procedures to enhance competitive performance were found. Of these seven, four met basic research design criteria. Of those four, none demonstrated significant performance-enhancing effects in competitive situations. Here again, another procedure widely thought to enhance performance demonstrated highly disappointing results.

Arousal Control

Five empirical studies utilized arousal control procedures (from relaxation to "psyching up") to enhance competitive athletic performance. Of these five, four met basic research design criteria, of which none resulted in significant performance-enhancing effects. This approach, while intuitively appealing as a performance-enhancement technique, therefore demonstrated troubling results upon careful examination.

Multicomponent Interventions

Frequently, empirical investigations include a number of PST procedures used in various combinations. Moore also examined empirical studies that utilized a "package" intervention approach including the above methods. Thirty-two studies using combinations of PST procedures for the purpose of competitive performance enhancement were found in the professional literature, and, of those 32, 12 met basic research criteria. Of those 12, 2 studies (both single-case multiple baseline studies published by the same author) using goal-setting, imagery, self-talk, and arousal control procedures demonstrated enhanced competitive performance. Separately, one study using self-talk and arousal control procedures suggested enhanced competitive performance. Another study of arousal control and imagery in 12- to 14-year-old competitive athletes resulted in significant performance improvements. Two additional studies using arousal control procedures (relaxation) and imagery resulted in performance enhancements. The other six studies that used multicomponent PST procedures demonstrated equivocal or no performance-enhancing effects. This suggests that the use of combined, or multicomponent, PST procedures are somewhat better than the use of individual procedures, but the inconsistency of the findings (6 of 12 studies resulted in performance enhancement) suggests that caution must be used and further suggests that the adoption of PST procedures as the gold standard of performance enhancement efforts is premature.

Potential explanations for these results include: (1) methodological problems in the studies (such as small sample sizes and inappropriate statistical procedures), making finding significant effects problematic; (2) assumptions regarding the homogeneity of athletes as a single, discreet population; (3) lack of clear theoretical connections between intervention methods and psychological processes related to optimal performance; (4) investigator allegiance effects; (5) inappropriate description of intervention protocols, thus reducing the generalizability and replicability of studies; and (6) poorly conceived and inappropriate measures of athletic performance. However, regardless of the reason for the disappointing results, one cannot deny a troubling lack of empirical support for these long-favored interventions. The fact remains that science places the burden of proof on those who make efficacy claims and not the critics who question efficacy claims (Lilienfeld, Lynn, & Lohr, 2003). Thus, while proponents of PST interventions may develop better ways of evaluating, measuring, or delivering psychological skills training procedures—and ultimately may produce the required efficacy studies—at present, the practitioner and public must carefully consider the implications of these findings.

At the heart of the true scientific method is the willingness to reevaluate and modify existing theory based on new scientific developments. Beyond the problematic lack of demonstrated efficacy noted above is concern regarding the theoretical appropriateness of PSTs for performance enhancement. The theoretical basis for the supposition that PST procedures can enhance human performance comes mainly from correlational studies, which have suggested that more successful performers are less anxious, more confident, and experience fewer negative thoughts than less successful ones (Gould, Eklund, & Jackson, 1992; Gould, Weiss, & Weinberg, 1981; Orlick & Partington, 1988). What has followed from these findings, and fundamental to the use of PSTs for performance enhancement, is the long-held assumption that reduction or control of negative thoughts, emotions, and bodily states and associated increases in confidence are directly related to the development of an "ideal performance state." This ideal performance state is, in turn, believed to lead to the desired outcome of optimal performance (Hardy et al., 1996). Further, it is assumed that, as interventions, PST procedures can effectively modify or control these internal processes.

In fact, the few studies that have evaluated the mechanisms of action (i.e., the variables that mediate the relationship between traditional PST procedures and competitive performance) of these procedures have generally not supported the basic assumptions that underlie these methods, thus calling into question the theoretical underpinning of such approaches. These studies, conducted across a variety of different sports, suggest that the reduction of negative emotions such as anxiety and increases in confidence do not consistently result in significant and meaningful increases in performance (Daw & Burton, 1994; Holm, Beckwith, Ehde, & Tinius, 1996; Maynard, Smith, & Warwick-Evans, 1995; Murphy & Wolfolk, 1987; Weinberg, Seaborne, & Jackson, 1981). Cohen, Pargman, and Tenenbaum (2003) completed a study in which experimentally manipulated levels of physiological arousal had no impact on competitive performance. Finally, a meta-analysis examining the role of confidence and competitive anxiety on athletic performance (Craft, Magyar, Becker, & Feltz, 2003) concluded that a weak relationship exists between anxiety, confidence, and performance. These empirical findings certainly suggest that intervention efforts aimed at the reduction of negative affective states, the reduction of negative thinking, and increases in confidence may have little significant impact on efforts to enhance performance.

Yet even if these variables are somehow related to the attainment of optimal performance states, the theoretical models underlying the common PST approaches have still failed to integrate many of the advances in the cognitive, clinical, and sport sciences over the past several decades. In light of the findings in Moore's review, questions regarding mechanisms of action, and failure to integrate advances from other psychology disciplines, it is reasonable to suggest that perhaps the theoretical models at the foundation of these PST procedures need to be reconsidered. By updating existing theories and developing new theoretical models for understanding functional and dysfunctional athletic performance (such as the IMHP presented in chapter 1), innovations in the use of psychological procedures for performance enhancement can be developed and systematically evaluated.

While readers are encouraged to access the comprehensive review (Gardner & Moore, 2006), the implications of these results for the practice of performance psychology are clear. Although it has not been demonstrated that these procedures do *not* work as advertised—because absence of evidence can never be interpreted as evidence of absence—the practitioner is nevertheless cautioned about enthusiastically adopting these procedures out of an assumption that these procedures *must* work because they have been traditionally utilized and because successful, respected professionals have frequently promoted their use.

We often provide our students and clients with a medical metaphor to make this point, by stating that long ago, well-respected and highly intelligent physicians used a procedure known as bloodletting to cure patients of medical ailments by withdrawing large amounts of blood from the patient. Of course, this procedure not only failed to cure patients of their ailments, it also killed many of them. So how does one answer these questions: (1) *Was the procedure a good one, meeting the needs of the client?* Clearly, the answer here is that the procedure was dangerous and did not meet the needs of the client. However, there was little way to know this until it was conducted and evaluated. (2) *Was the procedure wrong to do?* No, and maybe yes. The procedure was not wrong to do when bloodletting was considered to be the state-of-the-science medical practice. At one time, this procedure was cutting-edge and thoughtfully conceived based on existing evidence. It was probably better than previous methods, and it was abandoned as the state-of-the-science grew and new methods were available. However, the procedure would have been *wrong* to do if physicians maintained this practice using the guiding philosophy, "It's what we do," despite new scientific evidence determining its ineffectiveness. In essence, what we are saying here is that, despite more than 30 years of accumulated empirical findings, we do not have evidence that traditional PST procedures work to enhance performance. Should we continue to overlook these obvious findings, which are reinforced month after month when new journals publish the same findings, or should we turn to new scientific developments and advance past our comfort zone? When is it no longer okay to say, "It's what we do"?

MOVING ON: NEW INTERVENTION DIRECTIONS

In light of the absence of research demonstrating the efficacy of PST procedures and the absence of data to suggest that the mediating processes assumed to underlie PST procedures are related to optimal performance, the question for the practitioner is obvious. Where does one turn when seeking methods to enhance performance among clients? The answer begins by revisiting the Integrative Model of Human Performance. As presented in chapter 1, the IMHP suggests that interventions intended to enhance human performance should be individually tailored after careful assessment of the role of experiential avoidance and acceptance in self-regulatory disruption.

Over the past several years, an increasing body of literature has questioned the position that internal experiences judged to be negative invariably result in problematic behavioral outcomes (Hayes, Follete, & Linehan, 2004). Of particular relevance to performance psychology are findings suggesting that attempts to suppress or otherwise control unwanted thoughts and emotions can have a paradoxical effect. Suppression and control techniques can trigger a metacognitive scanning process that actively searches for signs of this unwanted cognitive-affective activity, bringing it to awareness when detected (Purdon, 1999; Wegner, 1994). The literature further suggests that efforts at thought suppression and control may also lead to more frequent unwanted thoughts and emotions (Clark, Ball, & Pape, 1991). When such unwanted thoughts are reactivated, the result is often an associated increase in emotional states and physiological arousal. Excessive cognitive activity and a task-irrelevant attentional focus replace task-relevant attention and goal-directed behavior. This disruption of the performance phase of the IMHP typically results in dysfunctional performance.

Conversely, empirical data (Barlow, 2002; Gardner & Moore, 2001; Rapee & Lim, 1992; Sbrocco & Barlow, 1996; Stopa & Clark, 1993) suggest that functional performance requires attention to external stimuli, options, and contingencies, often referred to as *task-focused attention.* This is in contrast to attention toward internal thoughts and processes, often referred to as *self-focused attention.* Thus, optimal human performance can be seen as requiring minimal self-judgment, minimal attention to external or internal threat, and minimal future-oriented focus on possible performance consequences and ramifications. This can be summarized as active absorption in the task as opposed to active absorption in the self.

Several studies have suggested the utility of this perspective in the context of performance psychology. Crocker, Alderman, and Smith (1988) utilized a stress-management intervention with elite volleyball players that included a meditation-like procedure aimed at developing the capacity to attend in-the-moment, as well as a coping skills package intended to develop one's capacity to focus on performance (task-focused attention) and cope with emotion. Interestingly, and theoretically consistent with acceptance-based predictions, there were nonsignificant reductions in anxiety and negative thoughts, yet there *were* significant performance improvements. These improvements were also maintained at 6-month follow-up. In addition, D'Urso, Petrosso, and Robazza (2002) conducted a qualitative analysis to assess the contribution of physical and psychological skills in a comparison between best and worst performances. The results suggested that psychological skills were not reliably related to performance differences, and, in fact, only physical skills were related in any significant way. The authors concluded "both positive and negative emotions may exert beneficial or detrimental effects, depending on their idiosyncratic meaning and intensity" (p. 172). This finding is also consistent with an acceptance-based theoretical position and would be predicted by the IMHP model.

To summarize, extant outcome and process/mediational data fail to support the intervention goals of reduction or control of negative affect, reduction or control of negative cognitive content, and increases in confidence levels in order to achieve enhanced performance. In fact, on both theoretical and empirical grounds, it can be argued that internal control-based approaches to performance enhancement (PST procedures) may inadvertently result in overly cognitive self-focused activity rather than the necessary task-focused and externally absorbed activity required to reach optimal performance states. Among other consequences, this may result in a reduced capacity to automatically engage in previously learned skills and abilities.

In response to the empirical and theoretical limitations associated with traditional PST procedures, and consistent with the theoretical and empirical foundations of the IMHP, we developed a new approach to performance enhancement called the Mindfulness-Acceptance-Commitment (MAC) approach (Gardner & Moore, 2004a, 2006).

MINDFULNESS-ACCEPTANCE-COMMITMENT (MAC) APPROACH

The Mindfulness-Acceptance-Commitment (MAC) approach to performance enhancement is an acceptance-based behavioral intervention designed specifically for use with performance populations. We developed the program specifically for performers after experiencing success with acceptance-based behavioral interventions in the clinical treatment room, after years of seeing athletes use traditional approaches to performance enhancement with no objective and sustainable performance improvements, and in response to the disappointing efficacy data for traditional performance enhancement procedures. In fact, acceptance-based approaches have garnered respect and success with clinical populations (Hayes, Follette, et al., 2004) and in nonclinical uses such as relationship enhancement (Carson, Carson, Gil, & Baucom, 2004), work-site stress reduction and performance enhancement (Bond & Bunce, 2000), and athletic performance enhancement (Gardner & Moore, 2004a, 2006; Wolanin, 2005).

On a theoretical level, this approach draws heavily upon the work of Hayes, Strosahl, and Wilson (1999), which suggests that, when an individual has an emotional response to an external stimulus—such as when one experiences anxiety during an important presentation or game—and then thinks about those situations at a later time, he or she is likely to experience anxiety directly to those thoughts. The actual (external) tasks, as well as the internal experiencing of the tasks (thoughts about the task), become cues for the emotion. This often results in excessive efforts to control one's internal experiences (thoughts or emotions) and/or overt efforts to avoid such experiences. In essence, although thoughts and emotions are simply passing subjective states, individuals often respond to their thoughts and emotions as though they are *realities* that need to be judged as good or bad, right or wrong, and acceptable or unacceptable. Such judgments subsequently guide one's choices and actions, which are frequently intended to avoid or escape those internal experiences judged to be negative, uncomfortable, or unacceptable. An example of this is the basketball player who becomes less aggressive, passes up open shots, and may even ask to be taken out of a game in response to the experience of anxiety or perseverative negative thoughts. As previously stated, Hayes and colleagues (1996) referred to this process as *experiential avoidance.* Anxiety, anger, or frustration experienced prior to an important meeting or competition may be associated with thoughts such as, "I'm too stressed to do this today," which, in turn, result in a decision to avoid the important event. In this example, the behavioral response directly guided by the individual's internal experience is an example of rule-governed behavior. In this case, the avoidant behavior is directly governed by the personal rule, "I can't handle meetings when I feel this bad" and is in direct response to the emotions and thoughts experienced. The avoidant behavior is not a choice or action that is in any way consistent with the valued goal of fully engaging in and enjoying the process of participation in one's chosen area of work.

To elucidate further, comments such as "I can't work for this guy; he's a jerk," or "I didn't take the shot because my confidence is down," reflect individuals who use their internal processes to explain and guide their behavioral choices. The behaviors that result from these internal "rules" are intended to reduce internal experiences such as frustration, anger, or anxiety (i.e., experiential avoidance). The affect-reduction function of these behaviors is in stark contrast to a more adaptive focus on valued behaviors, which may be contextually appropriate behaviors such as engaging in a meeting even when the client's boss has behaved badly and offended or upset the client, taking an open shot when available, working consistently to improve a skill, and experiencing the pain and boredom of injury rehabilitation. The distinction between rule-governed and values-directed behavior is critically important when one considers the fact that performers of all types and at all skill levels must regularly and consistently manage their behavior in the service of distal goals and at the expense of more immediate gratification. The MAC approach to performance enhancement is expected to promote both competitive in-the-moment behaviors as well as the values-directed behaviors necessary for practice, training, personal development, and development of elite skills.

The MAC approach promotes acceptance of one's internal experience, no matter what that might be, while at the same time focusing the performer on the contextually appropriate behavioral responses required to effectively navigate through life's ever-changing situations in order to fully engage in one's valued activities and achieve goals that really matter. Unlike more traditional approaches to performance enhancement that tend to focus primarily (and often solely) on competitive behaviors, the MAC approach promotes the enhancement of competitive behaviors and the decision-making, problem-solving, and behavioral processes involved in the client's day-to-day life. No performer is solely identified simply as a performer. Regardless of the performance domain, performers must also deal with other life issues. Some of these issues have nothing to do with the performance domain, and some indirectly affect competitive performance by impacting training, practice, and interpersonal relationships.

This discussion is intended to highlight the connection between the self-regulatory processes outlined in the IMHP and the theoretical rationale for the use of mindfulness, acceptance, and commitment-based concepts to enhance performance. As such, the MAC protocol described in a session-by-session manner later in this text targets the development of: (1) mindful, nonjudging, present-moment attention (mindfulness, to be discussed below); (2) acceptance of internal processes such as thoughts, emotions, and bodily sensations (as natural to the human experience); (3) a willingness to remain in contact with these internal experiences; and (4) a focus of attention on performance-relevant cues, contingencies, and situationally appropriate actions and choices in the service of personal performance and life values (commitment).

When achieved, the combination of processes targeted by MAC bear some basic similarities to the concept of flow often discussed in the sport and performance psychology literature (Csikszentmihalyi, 1990). It has been suggested that optimal performance requires the performer to achieve the outcome of present-moment, non–self-conscious concentration on a particular task. In his description of flow, Csikszentmihalyi (1990) described "the merging of action with awareness" (p. 53), "concentration on the task at hand" (p. 58), and "the loss of self-consciousness" (p. 62). Similarly, athletes have suggested that flow consists of seemingly automatic body movements, lack of awareness of thoughts and feelings, and heightened external awareness (Russell, 2001). All of these concepts are consistent with the goals of the MAC protocol.

As an innovative approach to performance enhancement, it is critical that the practitioner note that the development of mindful awareness, mindful attention, acceptance of internal processes, and task-appropriate, values-driven flexible behavior inherent in the MAC is intended to replace excessive efforts at internal self-control, task-irrelevant focus of attention, and restrictions in behavior that generally accompany less-than-optimal performance.

To further expand on the fundamental underpinning of the MAC approach, a major aspect of the MAC (and, in fact, all acceptance-based behavioral interventions) is the idea that a *flexible* approach to one's experiences—including thoughts, emotions, and bodily sensations—is essential for optimal functioning. In fact, an unwillingness to remain in contact with difficult internal experiences (experiential avoidance) is seen as a central factor leading to reduced behavioral functioning. This type of approach contrasts with classical cognitive-based intervention approaches, which essentially view emotional experiences as by-products of negative or "irrational" cognitive content (Beck, Emery, & Greenberg, 1985). From the traditional cognitive approach, people essentially feel the way they think, and, in turn, how people act is essentially a result of how they feel.

As an acceptance-based approach, the MAC takes a very different position:

> Instead of viewing control or reduction of internal experiences as a necessary means of creating the ideal performance state, the MAC approach emphasizes mindful, nonjudging awareness and acceptance of moment-to-moment cognitive, affective, and sensory experiences.

As humans, we never stop thinking, feeling, and experiencing bodily sensations. Yet, individuals are often told from a very young age that, for some reason, they should *not* experience some of these naturally occurring states and should work to minimize negative thoughts, try to hold back those tears, and ignore what their body is telling them. Despite efforts to suppress them, these experiences are naturally occurring events that, without fail, will regularly come and go as normal by-products of human existence. So, are they so bad? Are they wrong? Do they have to get in our way and hold so much power over us? According to recent conceptualizations of the beneficial role of emotion in human functioning, it is theorized that individuals who are able to stay in contact with their emotions (no matter what that emotion is) and can maintain full awareness of their emotional experience, understand the meaning of the emotion, utilize the information that comes from emotion, and manage the experience according to contextual realities can be expected to respond more effectively to performance and overall life demands. In this regard, the ability to attend to, process, and act upon emotional experiences in a manner that promotes one's valued goals has been termed *emotional intelligence* (Mayer, Salovey, & Caruso, 2004). Conversely, the effort to inhibit or otherwise avoid or limit the full experience of emotion has consistently been related to negative outcomes among studies in the clinical domain. For example, Lynch, Robins, Morse, and MorKrause (2001) found that emotional inhibition mediated the relationship between the intensity of emotion and psychological distress in both clinical and non-clinical samples. It was not the intensity of emotion per se that led to distress, but rather the degree to which individuals attempted to inhibit or avoid the emotional experience that was predictive of distress.

In addition, from an acceptance-based theoretical perspective, human difficulties also can be seen as evolving from the tendency of individuals to fuse with their cognitive processes (i.e., internal language) and thus view their thoughts, beliefs, and attitudes as absolute truths that provide reasons for events and, in turn, guide actions. Thus, rather than engaging in behaviors determined by the needs and realities of external cues and contingencies, behavioral choices are often guided by the belief that one's thoughts, emotions, and physical sensations require some immediate action. As a consequence, rather than making behavioral choices that reflect commitment to values that are personally meaningful—such as optimal performance (e.g., quality practice, aggressive competitive performance, maintenance of strategic plans under stress)—performance-related choices are made to avoid immediate discomfort and limit internal experiences judged to be unacceptable or uncomfortable. For example, the sales person who is having a difficult year is told that she needs to spend more time with potential new accounts. She becomes anxious when thinking about making cold calls and begins to think that she can't do it. She then contemplates what she would do if she lost her job, which results in sadness (at the thought of unemployment) and even more anxiety. She fuses with her self- and future-focused thought process, believes that thoughts of inability actually equal inability, and chooses to leave work early and call a friend to meet for drinks. This choice serves the immediate purpose of reducing the troubling internal processes and associated anxiety, and, as such, this avoidant behavior is negatively reinforced. However, this behavioral choice does nothing to improve sales performance, which requires consistent committed action regardless of uncomfortable internal experiences.

In the MAC, a great deal of attention is given to the acceptance-based concepts of willingness and commitment (Hayes et al., 1999). *Willingness* refers to the decision to fully experience thoughts, emotions, and sensations, regardless of whether they are pleasant. The willingness to fully experience life as it occurs allows the individual to have (accept) the full range of life, rather than to seek to avoid the inevitable uncomfortable moments that are part of being human. This willingness allows behavioral choices to be made not for the immediate relief of discomfort, but rather in the service of what is truly valued. *Commitment* can thus be defined as the process of actively choosing behaviors that are directly in pursuit of activities that enable the individual to pursue his or her personal values.

When discussing some of the concepts above, we frequently use terms such as *mindful awareness*. The development of *mindfulness* is a primary and central feature of MAC and, as such, deserves extended attention. Mindfulness can be seen as the process that promotes greater awareness of internal experiences and the defusion of one's thoughts, emotions, and bodily sensations as realities to which one must respond. As a process, mindfulness also can be viewed as a form of heightened present-moment awareness. It is a concept grounded in Eastern religious and philosophical traditions and has been defined as "paying attention in a particular way;

on purpose, in the present and nonjudgmentally" (Kabat-Zinn, 1994, p. 4). As a technique, mindfulness has been used as a component of numerous therapeutic interventions targeting a diverse array of clinical problems, such as borderline personality disorder, stress and anxiety, and recurrent depression (Kabat-Zinn, 1990; Linehan, 1993; Miller, Fletcher, & Kabat-Zinn, 1995; Roemer & Orsillo, 2002; Segal, Williams, & Teasdale, 2002). Mindful practice through a series of structured exercises and activities has been used in these interventions as a means of developing enhanced mindfulness as a *process* and has demonstrated a large body of empirical support (for a comprehensive review, see Baer, 2003).

Within the MAC approach to performance enhancement, mindfulness practice is conceptualized as a central core intervention that serves a variety of functions. In general, mindfulness techniques emphasize the development of nonjudging, nonevaluative attention to present realities, which include both external stimuli and internal processes, a central component of the IMHP. In essence, external and internal events that enter one's awareness are noticed but not evaluated as good, bad, right, wrong, helpful, or unhelpful. Individuals are taught to observe and describe, as opposed to judge and control, their experiences. Through this process:

> Mindfulness practice promotes mind*ful* responding as opposed to mind*less* reacting to life events.

Mindfulness also can be thought of as a basic attentional skill that is developed through regular practice of exercises, including a variety of meditation-inspired activities. With particular relevance to optimal performance, this skill can be viewed as a form of self-regulated present-moment attention (Kabat-Zinn et al., 1992) through its emphasis on noticing the full range of present-moment experiences. From a metacognitive perspective, mindfulness promotes greater attention to one's own attentional process and thus allows the individual to regulate how attentional processes are utilized (i.e., self- vs. task-focused attention).

In addition to promoting moment-to-moment attention, mindfulness-based techniques have also demonstrated efficacy in reducing the verbal-linguistic component of worry and anxiety (Roemer & Orsillo, 2002). As noted in chapter 1, a number of studies have confirmed that worry is characterized by a preponderance of cognitive activity and low levels of imagery and autonomic activity (Borkovec & Inz, 1990; Borkovec, Lyonfields, Wiser, & Deihl, 1993; Lyonfields, Borkovec, & Thayer, 1995). These findings are particularly important for those interested in performance enhancement given the recent findings in performance psychology, which suggest that elite performance is associated with decreased levels of left-hemisphere cortical activity, indicative of low levels of verbal-linguistic activity (Crews & Landers, 1993; Hatfield, Landers, & Ray, 1984; Janelle, Hillman, Apparies, et al., 2000; Janelle, Hillman, & Hatfield, 2000; Salazar, Landers, Petruzzello, & Han, 1990). Because increased cognitive activity has been shown to impede performance, there would seem to be a logical need to use *control*-based strategies to reduce cognitive activity. However, as we have discussed, control strategies require cognitive activity, and the added self-focus required by cognitive control strategies has been shown to have a paradoxical effect. In essence, direct efforts to minimize cognitive activity lead to *more* cognitive activity, thereby leading to performance impediments. Mindfulness strategies work much differently than control strategies and are able to achieve the goal of reduced activity without the paradoxical effect. This is one more reason that the MAC is a rational choice for use in efforts at performance enhancement.

To link mindfulness and the MAC approach, we suggest that mindfulness as a foundation to performance enhancement works through four basic processes. First, as an acceptance-based behavioral intervention, enhanced mindfulness promotes a primary goal of MAC, which is the reduction of efforts to exert control over private internal experiences such as thoughts, emotions, and physiological sensations. It is important to distinguish the promotion of acceptance of experience without any need to alter, control, fix, repair, or otherwise avoid life's experiences inherent in mindfulness practice from the change/control-based efforts common among traditional psychological skills training approaches. The reduction of efforts to control internal experiences is valuable for all types of clients, even performers experiencing intense recurring emotional reactions to performance situations. For such clients, mindfulness practice can even serve as a form of prolonged exposure to previously problematic and avoided thoughts, emotions, and physical sensations. Based on findings in contemporary learning theory that suggest that efforts to promote extinction of problematic affective responses must consider the context in which they occur (Bouton, 1993, 2002), it appears possible that the development of mindfulness skills may help establish an internal, and thus generalized, context that maintains the extinction of unwanted responses and may subsequently promote the acquisition of more adaptive behaviors. This is in contrast to traditional approaches to prolonged exposure that require very specific situational contexts, thus limiting the generalizability of the exposure procedures.

Second, the development of enhanced mindfulness positively influences the experience of emotion. Recent studies have suggested that mindfulness interventions can significantly increase the activation of the anterior region of the left hemisphere, which is associated with pleasant affect (Davidson et al., 2003). More specifically, it appears that mindfulness may alter the automatic behavioral responses that individuals develop around certain emotions. By changing the experience of emotion by allowing a given emotion to be fully embraced, individuals modify the behavioral responses that they had previously automatically demonstrated when experiencing those emotions. As such, the behaviors usually associated with problematic emotions—most typically manifesting in the form of avoidance—are altered and allow for more situationally appropriate and flexible behaviors. This would appear to be the likely outcome when individuals learn to observe, describe, and fully experience emotions without acting on them in any way. By doing so, the performer is better able to adaptively respond to the performance environment, rather than to his or her emotional states.

Third, based on the professional literature, mindfulness also operates through teaching individuals to see their own thoughts simply as thoughts and not absolute realities to which they must respond (Teasdale, Segal, & Williams, 1995; Wolanin, 2005). This has been referred to as metacognitive awareness (Teasdale et al., 1995), which is learning to observe a thought or emotion as just a thought or emotion and not an absolute reality that requires a response. In this regard, thoughts and emotions are seen simply as passing events that require no change or alteration. In contrast, when thoughts and feelings are seen as absolute realities that require immediate action, rule-governed behaviors are likely to occur. As previously noted, rule-governed behaviors reflect overgeneralized actions that are in response to strongly held internal rules instead of in response to situation-specific cues and contingencies. Rule-governed behaviors reflect specific behavioral patterns based on personal verbal rules that specify a direct relationship between actions (e.g., "When I give my closing argument to the jury . . .") and consequences (e.g., ". . . I will fail horribly and be laughed at"). Research has suggested that rule-governed behavior reduces an individual's sensitivity and ability to effectively respond to actual cues and contingencies in the environment (Hayes, Kohlenberg, & Melancon, 1989). From this perspective, the development of mindfulness does not, and is not intended to, reduce the frequency of distressing thoughts; nor does it in any way attempt to alter the content of one's thoughts. Rather, mindfulness serves to break down the literal belief in one's thoughts and internal rules. By doing so:

> Mindfulness enhances the individual's sensitivity to cues and contingencies in the environment and thus promotes greater behavioral flexibility.

Of added benefit, the breakdown of internal rules often includes freeing the individual from harsh and at times debilitating negative self-judgments.

Fourth, mindfulness aids the enhancement of human performance by promoting attentional focus onto necessary performance-relevant cues and contingencies instead of emotional stimuli and other internal processes. To achieve greater task-focused attention, mindfulness helps individuals focus on their attentional *process* and not simply on the object to which they are attending. One's attentional focus is therefore better able to shift as needed based on changing situational demands. Simply put, the development of mindfulness skills allows performers to focus attention on what they need to focus on as opposed to what they do not. In this regard, recent research has suggested that mindfulness is particularly effective in interrupting ruminative thoughts unrelated to the demands of the current moment (Teasdale et al., 1995). The relevance of enhanced self-regulation of attention processes can be seen in studies by Klinger, Barta, and Glas (1981) and Edwards, Kingston, Hardy, and Gould (2002), both of which suggest that the attentional shift from external game-related stimuli to internal self-evaluation of performance is a consistent and significant contributor to in-competition catastrophic performance decline in high performers. In addition, a recent study by Bogels, Sijbers, and Voncken (2006) suggests that a mindfulness-based task concentration protocol was effective in reducing self-focused attention, increasing task-focused attention, and reducing social performance anxiety, which is a form of performance dysfunction.

RESEARCH ON THE MAC PROTOCOL

As described, mindfulness and acceptance-based interventions have already accumulated research support for their use with a variety of populations. Yet, while the MAC approach to performance enhancement is largely comprised of these empirically informed approaches, it is still necessary to conduct studies on the efficacy of the MAC approach to performance enhancement. In contrast to the empirical evidence that indicates a troubling lack of efficacy for traditional psychological skills training procedures for the enhancement of performance enhancement, there is a growing body of empirical data suggesting that the MAC can be effective in enhancing performance (Gardner & Moore, 2004a, 2006; Gardner, Wolanin, & Moore, 2005; Lutkenhouse, Gardner, & Morrow, 2007; Wolanin, 2005).

A study conducted in 2003 investigated the efficacy of the preliminary version of the MAC protocol (Wolanin, 2005). Eleven Division I collegiate athletes participated in the MAC program and were compared to seven matched control subjects. Results indicated that athletes receiving the MAC protocol manifested significant improvements on self- and coach ratings of performance compared to control subjects. In addition, self- and coach ratings of concentration and aggressiveness also significantly improved compared to controls.

A substantially larger trial ($N = 118$) recently conducted by Lutken- house and colleagues (2007) investigated the performance enhancement effects of the MAC approach compared to a traditional psychological skills training intervention protocol. Three Division I collegiate athletic teams (men's soccer = 26; women's soccer = 17; and women's field hockey = 17; total $N = 60$) participated in the weekly seven-session MAC pro- tocol. The MAC intervention group was compared to three, equivalent- level Division I collegiate teams (men's wrestling = 30; men's crew = 14; women's crew = 14; total $N = 58$) that received a weekly seven-session psychological skills training protocol used by the United States Olympic Committee (USOC; 1999). The published USOC protocol utilizes goal- setting, imagery, relaxation/stress-management, positive self-talk, and energy management/arousal control procedures. These six teams were randomly assigned to the intervention condition; each intervention was delivered to individual teams in a group format. No significant differ- ences were noted at pretest between the two groups on any athlete or coach ratings of performance. Results indicate that an equal number of individuals in each group showed some improvements in coach ratings of performance from pre- to posttest. However, a significantly greater number of athletes completing the MAC protocol demonstrated a clini- cally significant increase (at least a 20% improvement) on coach ratings of performance at posttest (32% of MAC participants compared to 10% of PST participants; Chi-Square = 6.2, $df = 1$, $p < .03$). In addition, the MAC group demonstrated significant posttest increases in aggressive- ness ($p < .01$) with a corresponding reduction in experiential avoidance ($p < .03$) and increase in flow scores ($p < .05$).

When evaluating the mechanisms by which the MAC protocol is hypothesized to enhance performance (reduced experiential avoidance, enhanced mindful awareness, enhanced mindful attention, and enhanced "flow"), the MAC group demonstrated significant pre-post improve- ments and also demonstrated significantly greater improvements than the PST group in the reduction of experiential avoidance (Acceptance and Action Questionnaire; $p < .01$), absorption in task (Flow Scale; $p < .04$), and mindful awareness/attention (Cognitive and Affective Mindfulness Scale; $p < .01$).

These studies provide support for the hypothesis that the integration of mindfulness techniques and acceptance-based behavioral procedures can be effectively applied to performers seeking to attain optimal performance levels. The data from these studies suggest that the use of MAC results in increased objective measures of performance and increased coach ratings of enhanced performance. In addition, as predicted by the theoretical foundation of the MAC approach, performers whose performance was effectively enhanced demonstrated: (1) increases in ratings of concentration and aggressive/nonavoidant performance behavior; (2) increases in mindful attention and awareness; (3) self-reported reductions in both believability of negative thoughts and the use of avoidance as a general behavioral strategy; and (4) enhanced levels of "flow" during performance tasks.

CONCLUSION

In recent years, mindfulness and acceptance-based approaches to understanding behavioral difficulties have emerged in the clinical science literature and have begun to change the nature of behavioral interventions for a variety of client difficulties. This chapter has presented the theoretical and empirical rationale for the development of an innovative intervention for the enhancement of performance. The Mindfulness-Acceptance-Commitment approach to performance enhancement is based on an integration of mindfulness and acceptance-based approaches and is specifically tailored for high-performing clientele.

The theoretical and empirical foundation of MAC described and discussed in this chapter should be an ongoing reference for practitioners who wish to utilize this approach. The effective use of the MAC approach requires that the practitioner question, and even alter, many long-held views about performance enhancement. It has been our experience that the successful utilization of the MAC intervention requires the practitioner to both understand and embrace the theoretical model (to avoid inadvertently conveying mixed messages) and to engage in personal efforts at using these principles and techniques in one's own life. As a practitioner, your personal utilization of mindfulness practice, acceptance of internal experiences, and commitment to values-driven behavior will allow you to both understand and empathize with your clients' experiences in the course of their journey through the MAC protocol.

The MAC approach to performance enhancement will be presented in detail as we describe the entire session-by-session protocol in part II. However, before embarking upon the MAC protocol, chapter 3 introduces a way of understanding and classifying performers' needs that will bridge the theoretical framework presented in chapters 1 and 2 with an understanding of the particular interventions most helpful in ameliorating the vast array of performance barriers.

CHAPTER 3

Planning for the MAC

The professional practice of performance psychology requires a conceptually sound and evidence-based integration of assessment and intervention designed to provide high-level care to the individuals who desire such services. This chapter describes a systematic approach to intervention planning in performance psychology. The model of intervention planning presented here is based on the case formulation method for sport psychology we have described elsewhere (Gardner & Moore, 2005) and provides a framework for understanding the performer and the myriad of issues that he or she brings to the consulting room. Based on the IMHP theoretical model presented in chapter 1, this case formulation method allows an individually tailored MAC intervention to be developed for each client.

CONCEPTUALIZING THE PERFORMER

In the case formulation method suggested in this chapter, the practitioner's first goal is to conceptualize performance needs and barriers based on the information systematically collected during the assessment process. This conceptualization should include the following:

- A comprehensive evaluation of the presenting problem, which allows for careful consideration of the environmental or situational triggers; dispositional variables; problematic cognitive, emotional, and behavioral responses; and maintaining factors.
- An understanding of the psychological and behavioral processes that emanate from and are directly linked to the referral issue. The consultant must understand that the MAC does not directly target outcomes. Rather, the MAC targets *processes* that

41

are directly related to optimal performance and that ultimately result in desired performance outcomes. The professional literature often refers to these processes as "mechanisms of action" (Barlow et al., 2004).

Assessing the Athlete

The consultant begins the case formulation process by engaging in a comprehensive biopsychosocial assessment of the client. The answers to the following questions, posed during the assessment process, guide the case formulation method:

- What are the presenting issues, how did these issues develop, and what factors trigger and maintain these issues?
- What are the situational and performance demands of the client?
- What are the skill requirements of the client's performance area, and what is the client's personal development in this area?
- What is the performer's current skill level?
- What are the performer's performance schemas (including attitudes and expectations about performance and personal rules regarding effort, success, mistakes, failure, etc.)?
- What thoughts, emotions, and behavioral responses characterize varying aspects of the client's performance?
- To what degree does the client focus on performance cues and contingencies, and to what degree does he or she focus on self and performance ramifications during actual performance?
- How does the client respond to performance setbacks?
- To what degree (and when) does the client worry, ruminate, procrastinate, or employ other forms of experiential avoidance?
- What work-related, sport-related, or personal performance learning experiences contribute to current performance concerns?
- What are the current stressors and physical circumstances that contribute to the presenting issues?
- What is the performer's cognitive and behavioral coping style in response to these issues, and how do the presenting issues affect his or her view of the self, others, and the future?

All of these questions must be asked and answered during the assessment process. The case formulation method is intended to be systematic, comprehensive, and holistic. Both during and after assessment, the information gathered needs to be organized so that it provides a larger picture of the performer's presenting complaints, leads to an appropriate classification (discussed later in this chapter), and culminates in an individualized MAC intervention plan. We will now briefly review some of the assessment strategies that may be used in collecting the information necessary for a comprehensive case formulation.

Assessment Strategies

The three primary strategies for information collection in professional psychology are the interview, behavioral observation, and psychological testing. Combined, these elements typically are referred to as *psychological assessment*. When performed correctly, these three strategies can be seamlessly integrated to determine prognosis, direct the selection and implementation of an appropriate intervention strategy, and reasonably predict the outcome.

Interview

The most common form of assessment in professional psychology is the interview. The earliest form of interview was based on the assumption that the information required for understanding personal difficulties and dynamics can be ascertained through an unstructured meeting that allows clients to freely discuss personal information that they deem relevant. This type of interview required little direction from the consultant. However, the natural subjectivity inherent in the unstructured interview and the desire for more objective and reliable means of collecting information led to the development of semistructured and structured interview formats and promoted the use of a myriad of psychological tests (First, Spitzer, Gibbon, & Williams, 1997).

The unstructured interview tends to be unreliable, because it is procedurally inconsistent, subject to clinician biases, and lacks empirical validation (Groth-Marnat, 1999). The subjective dangers inherent in the unstructured interview, which by definition relies on the interviewer's clinical judgment, are most clearly noted in a meta-analysis by Grove and colleagues (Grove, Zald, Lebow, Snitz, & Nelson, 2000). Their comprehensive review of the professional literature found that mechanical prediction of human behavior (using statistically derived scales and formulas) was consistently more accurate than clinical judgment (predictions made by subjectively evaluating test or interview data) in nearly all of the 136 studies comparing the two approaches. Interestingly and of great significance, they found that clinical interpretations of objective test data become less accurate when the clinician has interview data at his or her disposal (Grove et al., 2000). These findings indicate that the consultant engaging in unstructured interviews must take great care when drawing subjective conclusions about clients' (including performers') issues. The unstructured interview without goal-directed aims or psychometric data can quickly dissolve into a likeability contest in which the practitioner makes inferences based on the overall *feeling* he or she has about the client. Variables such as the performer's personal appearance, ethnicity, history, attitude, and belief system can impact the practitioner's interpretation of the performer's presenting issues, etiology, and likely intervention needs. The comprehensive review by Grove et al. (2000) reinforces the need for objective assessment, including both inventories (psychological tests) and semistructured or structured interview formats.

While numerous practitioners have called for inventories and other objective methods to be integrated into the work of the performance psychologist (Gardner, 1995; Gordin & Henschen, 1989; Nideffer & Sagal, 2001; Perna, Neyer, Murphy, Ogilvie, & Murphy, 1995), others have proposed that using inventories and other semistructured or structured assessment approaches is unnecessary or even detrimental to their work (Dorfman, 1990; Halliwell, 1990; Orlick, 1989; Ravizza, 1990; Rotella, 1990). From their perspective, informal interviews that are consistent with the practitioner's personal style and practice philosophies allow information to be collected in an atmosphere that is nonthreatening and reportedly more accepted by performers. This point of view has been stressed especially in the athletic domain, where some practitioners believe that athletes will oppose direct questioning, the use of assessment measures, or any element that makes the atmosphere seem too clinical. While the unstructured interview style does promote a comfortable atmosphere, there are clear dangers in making decisions based on personal style, beliefs, or philosophies. The proposition that experience and professional judgment are both necessary and sufficient to make important professional decisions is inconsistent with the data and unacceptable to an evidence-based practice of performance psychology. The data regarding clinical judgments are clear, and a legitimate evidence-driven profession cannot ignore such findings based on anecdotal reports and personal opinion alone.

In response to the dangers of the unstructured interview, semistructured and structured interviews (First et al., 1997) have become popular among professional psychologists and have been shown to be both reliable and valid indicators of client concerns. One particular interview, the Sport-Clinical Intake Protocol (SCIP), is an example of a structured interview for sport psychology (Taylor & Schneider, 1992). The SCIP focuses on both sport and nonsport issues and allows for comprehensive and consistent data collection with face-to-face collaborative client interaction. The SCIP interview clearly demonstrates that semistructured or structured interviews do not inherently create an artificial or noncol-laborative atmosphere.

We have developed a semistructured interview based on the Multi-level Classification System for Sport Psychology (MCS-SP; discussed later in this chapter). Although the MCS-SP (Gardner & Moore, 2004b) and the associated interview were originally designed for the comprehensive assessment and classification of athletes' issues and needs, the classifi-cation system and interview are fully appropriate for any performance issues presented to the psychologist. The MCS-SP semistructured inter-view can greatly assist the assessment process and help clarify presenting issues, which inevitably assists case formulation and intervention efforts. The format of this interview is not intended to be static or sequential. We recommend that consultants wishing to incorporate this interview into their practice approach the interview questions as a guide for sound data collection. Instead of asking rote and mechanical questions that challenge a sound therapeutic bond, the consultant can be conversational through-out the interview by collecting information during the natural ebb and flow of the consultant-client interaction.

Although not a formal interview, a particular style of semistructured interview that we highly value is the functional analysis of behavior (Hayes et al., 1996) (described later in this chapter). This type of interview style does not suggest a specific, structured set of questions to ask the cli-ent in a specific order. Instead, during the collaborative interchange with the client, the practitioner inquires about the "who," "what," "when," "where," "why," "how," and "how much" relating to the client's present-ing issue or problem. Why is this important? Most readers will be very knowledgeable about how to diagnose a client. Yet diagnosis requires a fairly superficial, yes-or-no answer to a variety of symptom complaints. For example, to diagnose major depressive disorder, the practitioner as-sesses a variety of common characteristics associated with depression, such as changes in appetite and sleep patterns, lethargy/fatigue, and dif-ficulty concentrating. Having this information enables the practitioner to definitely say that the client meets or does not meet the criteria for major depressive disorder. Yet does the practitioner really *know* the client based on this information? If the practitioner described the client's symptoms to another person, could that person form a complete and accurate picture of the client and his or her dysfunction? Certainly not. The functional analysis, on the other hand, allows the practitioner to supplement and clarify this diagnostic information, to gather the pertinent information that *surrounds* the diagnosis. For example, the functional analysis will tell the practitioner about triggers, subtle consequences (reinforcers) of behaviors, maintaining factors, what makes the problem better and worse, secondary gain, the role of relationships, and so on. In essence, the functional analysis explicates relevant target behaviors, triggers, and factors that maintain specific behaviors needing reduction or augmentation. This type of information allows the practitioner to personalize any diagnostic information and see the real person underlying the concerns. With the goal of obtaining such a breadth and depth of information, the functional analysis is at the heart of a comprehensive case formulation, including the MCS-SP semistructured interview.

The interview process may also benefit from the active participation of family members, management/coaching personnel, and other relevant parties when appropriate and with full client approval and written consent. This participation is often essential to comprehensively understanding the problem context and typically ensures that the critical people in the performer's life both support and understand the services to be provided.

Behavioral Observation

The second primary strategy in the assessment process is directly observing client behavior, which can occur in several contexts. First, the consultant may have the opportunity to directly observe the client within his or her performance context. Particularly when working with athletes and musicians, the consultant may attend competition or practice. The consultant can then directly observe interpersonal interactions; verbal and nonverbal responses to both good and bad performances; body language in response to manager, coach, or referee decisions; and similar types of overt behavior along with antecedent events and consequent behavior. These observations allow the consultant to create a real-life context for the words and descriptions the performer provides in private sessions.

Second, and perhaps most importantly, behavioral observations are inherent within the interview itself. The consultant should note a performer's response to frustrating questions or inventories, behavior when anxious or angry, and similar reactions. Why should these reactions be so different than reactions displayed in other contexts outside the consultation room? In this regard, we teach the novice clinicians we supervise that the client's in-session behavior is essentially a small sample of what the client experiences outside of the session. These reactions yield critical information about the client's internal and external experience. Whatever the context, directly observing behavior provides the consultant useful information to integrate into the assessment process. However, behavioral observations are most useful when described objectively and when the consultant limits subjective interpretation of behaviors and responses until he or she has collected all of the relevant data. For example, the consultant observing that an athlete rolled her eyes each time her coach criticized her is significantly more objective than the consultant witnessing the action and subjectively concluding that the response represents oppositional and defiant behavior. The latter is more judgmental and evaluative and may lead to data misinterpretation. Although the consultant's interpretation may be true, early subjective interpretation can cloud the consultant's judgment and may lead to confirmatory bias. Thus, we recommend objective description of behavioral observations and suggest withholding interpretation of behavioral data until sufficient data have been collected.

Behavioral observations should be integrated into the case formulation in the context of all the data collected. Certainly, the most important observations are those behaviors directly relating to the presenting issues. The professional literature refers to observed (in-session) behavior directly relevant to the presenting issue as *clinically relevant behavior* (Kohlenberg & Tsai, 1995).

Psychological Testing

Psychological testing, often referred to as psychometric evaluation, is the third common assessment strategy. There are several basic recommendations for using psychometric instruments in the context of performance psychology. To ethically and effectively use data from psychological inventories or tests, consultants should understand that individual scores derived from these instruments are not end products, but rather are additional data points in the assessment process that allow hypotheses to be generated, confirmed, or disconfirmed. The data obtained from assessment instruments should be integrated with information from other assessment strategies (such as semistructured interviews and behavioral observations) to form a comprehensive whole. Considerable evidence supports the use of psychological testing in organizational contexts for purposes not unlike those found in performance psychology (Hogan, Hogan, & Roberts, 1996). While useful for the collection of necessary information, when determining how psychological testing will be integrated into the assessment process, the consultant should consider a variety of factors, including construct validity of the test in the context of the referral question, reliability, standardization of the instrument, and practical considerations such as time and availability.

CASE FORMULATION

Following the collection of all necessary information, the consultant needs to organize and synthesize these data into a comprehensive whole.

There are 10 elements of our comprehensive case formulation approach (Gardner & Moore, 2005); in general, after eliciting the presenting problem or reason for referral, developing useful case formulation requires a careful consideration of these 10 basic elements:

1. Contextual performance demands
2. Current performance-relevant skill development
3. Relevant situational demands (including performance and nonperformance demands)
4. Transitional and developmental issues
5. Unique psychological characteristics: performance and non-performance schemas
6. Direction of attentional focus (self versus task) during performance
7. Cognitive responses
8. Affective responses
9. Behavioral responses
10. Readiness for change and level of reactance

The first three elements include contextual performance demands, personal skill development, and the situational demands faced by the performer. These three separate but interrelated elements must be carefully considered, regardless of whether the client is an individual or an entire group (such as a sales team or athletic team). *Contextual performance demands* refer to the performer's level of competitive or work-related activity and the performance demands that are inherent to that activity. The demands of professional sports greatly differ from the demands of an entry-level salesperson, which in turn differs from the demands of a junior-level executive, and so on. In addition, each performer is likely to report a different personal experience than a coworker or teammate who is in the same environment and has the same performance demands.

Contextual performance demands intersect with the performer's *skill level* to affect performance in a highly individualized way. Performer's skills are usually developed to the level where they can generally handle the contextual performance demands they face. For instance, a Division I freshman point guard (with the characteristic skill sets of a Division I freshman) can perform at her expected level, and thus experiences an appropriate intersection between contextual performance demands and level of skill. When adding *relevant situational demands,* the intersection will take a unique shape. Using the previous example, a situational demand would be placing the freshman point guard into a starting role following a teammate's unexpected injury. Clearly, the performer will face a different set of performance demands than she is used to under normal circumstances. Depending on the performance domain, there are obviously a wide variety of possible situational demands that may affect performance, such as working for a company experiencing serious financial difficulties, a modified role on a team due to injury, challenges to an executive's interpersonal fit within the organization following a corporate merger, and so on.

For the most part, the first three elements are assessed through an interview format and may or may not be aided by the integration of information collected from outside sources such as family members, teammates, or coaches/managers.

The next element of the case formulation method is *transitional and developmental issues.* This refers to the developmental issues and milestones that are experienced by all humans as a natural part of life. Transitional and developmental issues refer to situations that typically occur within defined periods of life and include psychosocial stressors that unexpectedly but nevertheless naturally occur throughout life. Examples include transitioning in and out of college, early career stress, mid- or late career issues, retirement (chosen or forced), injury, financial stress, illness or disability, marriage and family concerns, loss of a loved one, and relationship difficulties. Each of these concerns will have significant personal meaning to the client and will likely impact performance. Thus, they should be carefully considered in the context of the client's performance issues and concerns. Of course, concerns such as these are often unpredictable or evolutionary in nature. We suggest that the consultant take the advice of Cates (1999), who suggested that assessment should not be seen as a snapshot, but instead should be viewed as a film. In essence, since concerns such as these come and go, assessment can never truly be complete. It is essential to occasionally reassess not only the client's performance concerns, but also the life issues that may be negatively affecting both performance and general life domains.

The next element requiring consideration is the performer's unique *psychological characteristics,* which may be made up of performance and nonperformance schemas. As discussed earlier in this text, schemas are internal rule systems developed over time that form the template by which individuals appraise and interpret their world (Gardner & Moore, 2006; Young, Klosko, & Weishaar, 2003). Within performance domains, common schemas may take the form of extreme perfectionism, self-perceptions of inadequacy, the need to please others, and fear of failure. Schemas can also be unrelated to performance, such as viewing oneself as unlovable; feeling inherently vulnerable; and believing that abandonment, rejection, and disappointment will inevitably occur. Psychological characteristics such as these are not only critical to assess in and of themselves, but also because they inevitably affect the intersection of the first three elements noted earlier. Personal psychological factors may also include other psychological processes such as worry, rumination, and experiential avoidance, to name a few.

While the interview process is likely to result in hypotheses regarding individual psychological characteristics, it is in this area that the use of psychological testing is most helpful. Within professional psychology, a number of brief psychometric measures have been developed that effectively target specific psychological characteristics. For example, the Young Schema Questionnaire (Young, 1999, 2002) has been developed to identify early maladaptive schemas that can impact both performance and overall life functioning. Other measures have been developed for a variety of specific psychological characteristics. To name a few, the Frost Multidimensional Perfectionism Scale (Frost, Marten, Lahart, & Rosenblate, 1990) measures perfectionism, the Penn State Worry Questionnaire (Meyer, Miller, Metzger, & Borkovec, 1990) assesses worry, and the Action and Acceptance Questionnaire-Revised (Hayes, Strosahl, Wilson, Bissett, et al., 2004) measures experiential avoidance. A complete review and compilation of all these measures is well beyond the scope of this text, but readers are encouraged to learn more about these important targeted psychological tests (Gardner & Moore, 2006).

As noted in chapter 1, the integration of the client's performance history and psychological characteristics intersects with situational demands and skill level to set the stage for functional or dysfunctional competitive activity. For example, consider the client whose core performance schema involves personal competence that often results in dysfunctional levels of perfectionism. If this client is required to work for a new supervisor who is overly demanding and interpersonally abrasive, she is likely to respond to performance demands much differently than when she previously worked for a supportive and pleasant supervisor. The performance demands should be seen within the context of the performer's underlying psychological characteristics (relentless perfectionism) and the situational changes (punitive and challenging new supervisor). Because every referral has a unique interaction between external demands and personal characteristics, the consultant should carefully examine this interaction before intervening. In this example, if the consultant overlooks the presence of dysfunctional perfectionism that is underlying the performance issue, the consultant may decide that traditional self-talk strategies will help the client maintain her focus and adjust to the new environment. This would clearly be a big mistake. However, the consultant who recognizes the performance schema and the presence of extreme perfectionism will know (if aware of the scientific literature) that, under such circumstances, cognitive strategies such as self-talk are likely to exacerbate the problem.

Understanding the client's psychological characteristics is a step that cannot be overlooked or devalued. Once the consultant has determined the client's relevant psychological characteristics, he or she can identify the sixth element in the case formulation approach, which is the performer's direction of *attentional focus* (self versus task) during performance. To assess this important element, we suggest that the consultant answer the following questions:

- Are the performer's thoughts self-referenced or task appropriate?
- Does the performer focus on the present moment during work/competition, or is his or her focus of attention on the possibility of failure, personal concerns, or unrelated events?
- Is the performer angry or anxious, or frustrated, and, if so, does he or she view experiencing these emotions as problematic?
- Do efforts at monitoring or controlling internal experiences such as thoughts or emotions predominate over focus on performance-related external cues and contingencies?

Why is determining the performer's attentional focus so important? As noted in chapter 1, empirical data indicate that task-focused attention is critical to functional human performance, and, conversely, excessive self-focused attention is strongly related to dysfunctional performance in sport, sexual, and academic domains (Barlow, 2002; Gardner & Moore, 2004a, 2006; Harvey, Watkins, Mansell, & Shafran, 2004). Given this knowledge, the consultant should carefully assess this important dimension. Related to the concept of attentional direction is the concept of self-awareness, which is the degree to which the performer is aware of his or her internal events (cognitions and emotions), and external processes (behavior). The professional literature strongly suggests that this combination of attention and awareness is related to both positive performance outcomes and personal well-being.

The seventh, eighth, and ninth elements of the case formulation method are separate but interrelated elements that include the performer's cognitive, affective, and behavioral responses to both performance and nonperformance stimuli. *Cognitive responses* refer to the specific cognitive content or automatic thoughts that are experienced during performance-related activities. This variable reflects what clients report they tell themselves during performance-relevant situations. An important consideration here is whether performers view their thoughts as absolute facts that accurately represent reality or as ideas that simply come and go, which may require a response when necessary, may deserve an outright dismissal, or may simply be seen as random and passing experiences. Recent research suggests that it is not the content of the thoughts that is related to psychological and behavioral difficulties (i.e., negative or positive thoughts), but, rather, it is the degree to which an individual *believes* that his or her thoughts are real or factual that predicts behavioral difficulties (Hayes et al., 1999). In essence, the more the performer believes in the absolute, factual nature of his or her (negative) thoughts, the greater the likelihood that these thoughts will in some way interfere with performance. Cognitive content can be easily determined via a semistructured interview.

The performer's *affective responses* are triggered by performance-related situations. This category refers to the typical emotions that are experienced by the performer in the course of his or her performance life. Questions to consider include:

- Does the performer frequently experience anxiety, frustration, or anger in response to work/competitive situations?
- Does the performer believe that these emotions are in some way related to either positive or negative performances?
- Is the performer's characteristic style of emotion processing healthy (brief expression of contextually appropriate emotion) or unhealthy (overutilization of experiential avoidance to regulate negative affect)?

While affective responses are often linked to cognitive responses, it is important to independently evaluate and record each as individual processes. Affective processes can be readily ascertained via interview and with the use of a number of brief psychometric measures (Gardner & Moore, 2006).

Finally, we are interested in understanding the performer's *behavioral responses* to the work/competitive situation. Such behavioral responses commonly will be characteristic of behavioral response patterns demonstrated in other life domains. Typical behavioral responses span from the active coping and activation of behaviors necessary for improvement and success to avoidance and the associated effort to reduce, eliminate, or otherwise control difficult or uncomfortable internal experiences. This element is particularly important, because overt behavior leads most performers to seek consultation. Whether the goal is to further develop performance, reduce responses to situational factors that are impeding necessary work/competitive behavior, or reduce worry and task avoidance, carefully reviewing referral questions in all domains of professional psychology leads to the unmistakable conclusion that clients ultimately want to *function* (behave) more efficiently or effectively. Enhanced behavioral functioning can take the form of optimal work/competitive performance, better parenting skills, better responses to frustration, and enhanced interpersonal relationships. While *feeling better* is often thought to be required for enhanced functioning, the MAC program suggests that improved functioning can occur *despite* feeling badly. For example, the athlete who is angry with his coach or teammate or who is sad over the breakup of a significant relationship can nevertheless function by remaining focused on the cues and contingencies required for athletic competition. Achieving this focus requires the capacity to decenter (step back and self-observe), and a willingness to have uncomfortable internal experiences, and an ability to resist engaging in efforts to gain immediate emotional relief. Defining the behavior in need of modification is the most rational means of understanding the performer's current performance functioning and designing an individually tailored MAC protocol that directly targets that functioning.

The tenth and final element in the case formulation process is the evaluation of the performer's readiness for change and level of reactance, both of which are related to intervention efficacy in the clinical psychology literature (Blatt, Shahal, & Zurhoff, 2002). *Readiness for change* is a central concept in the transtheoretical model of behavior change presented by Prochaska, DiClemente, and Norcross (1992) and reflects attitudes and behaviors regarding the need for and commitment to behavior change. An individual's readiness for change reflects a number of interacting variables, including motivation, expectancy, efficacy, and openness to assistance (Burke, Arkowitz, & Menchola, 2003). Considering these variables may help the practitioner determine the need for enhancing the performer's readiness for change before beginning more active or structured interventions. Measures such as the Readiness for Change Questionnaire may help in this regard (Forsberg, Halldin, & Wennberg, 2003). *Reactance* has received research attention as a potential moderator that may selectively predict a client's response to different psychological interventions. Reactance has been defined as a motivational state characterized by the client's tendency to restore or reassert his or her abilities and freedoms when he or she perceives that they are lost or being threatened by others (Beutler, Consoli, & Williams, 1995). The highly reactant individual has been described as "dominant," "individualistic," and "oppositional" (Dowd, Milne, & Wise, 1991; Dowd, Wallbrown, Sanders, & Yesenosky, 1994) and is likely to be reactive or oppositional when faced with external efforts at influencing behavior (Beutler & Consoli, 1993). The characteristics noted in this definition can frequently be found in highly successful individuals and as such should be carefully considered in the case formulation method. Beutler, Consoli, and Williams (1995) and others (Dowd et al., 1994) have suggested that reactance is an important variable to consider during intervention planning, because it is likely to predict client resistance to directive intervention methods. The consultant should carefully assess this variable during the semistructured interview process, because the empirical evidence suggests that early intervention efforts should be less directive for clients high in reactance (Beutler et al., 1995) to help prevent premature termination.

CLASSIFYING PERFORMANCE ISSUES

With all 10 of the basic elements necessary for a comprehensive case formulation fully understood, the consultant is ready to correctly classify the client's performance issues and concern based on the Multilevel Classification System for Sport Psychology (MCS-SP). This classification system was originally designed to classify athletes' concerns and issues, yet is equally functional at determining relevant barriers holding back performers of all types. It is only following the appropriate MCS-SP classification that the MAC program should be initiated, because individuals of different MCS-SP classifications may respond differently to various elements of the MAC protocol. What follows is a description of the MCS-SP.

Research in sport and performance psychology has typically designed performance enhancement intervention studies with the underlying assumption that individuals seeking to improve performance are inherently psychosocially well functioning and possess essentially homogeneous personal characteristics and intervention needs (Vealey, 1994). Because of this pattern, performers are rarely differentiated by psychological and behavioral factors beyond their most obvious performance needs, and consultants are usually left with no systematic way of determining which type of intervention is appropriate for which client. Unfortunately, this pattern has subsequently led to one-size-fits-all approaches to intervention.

Thus, in response to the absence of a clear, systematic, and comprehensive classification system within performance psychology, we developed the Multilevel Classification System for Sport Psychology for assessing, conceptualizing, and classifying issues frequently seen by practicing sport and performance psychologists (Gardner & Moore, 2004b). The MCS-SP suggests a clear and logical decision-making process for client assessment and intervention planning.

The MCS-SP categorizes the issues and barriers facing the performer into four classifications: performance development (PD), performance dysfunction (Pdy), performance impairment (PI), and performance termination (PT).

Performance Development

The performance development classification represents issues brought to the performance consultant in which:

- A desire to improve performance is stated as the primary reason for seeking of consultation.
- There is an absence of significant transitional, behavioral, developmental, intrapersonal, or interpersonal psychological factors affecting performance or requiring attention.
- Developing and/or refining psychological skills will likely enhance performance.

There are two subtypes within the PD category. PD-I refers to cases in which mental skills may be helpful to promote ongoing development of necessary performance skills and/or to enhance work/competitive performance. For performers of this type, skill development is underway but is not yet complete. PD-II clients have already developed a high level of necessary skills, and the development of mental skills is indicated to attain consistently higher-level performance.

The overall goal in the performance development category is the direct enhancement of performance. To obtain this classification, the consultant must determine through the interview and assessment process that the performer's psychological functioning is adequate and that the client desires a realistic level of performance or performance consistency that he or she has yet to attain or demonstrate consistently. The consultant should also carefully assess for developmental, transitional, intrapersonal, interpersonal, or clinical issues affecting the performer, because such issues warrant a different classification.

The typical PD performer is a reasonably well-functioning client who would like to further develop his or her performance-related skills and performance consistency to reach a realistically high level of overall performance. Such clients typically want to learn how to more effectively utilize their psychological and behavioral processes to reach this goal. The PD classification also includes performers who exhibit inconsistent performance and who experience relatively short-term yet persistent decrements (slumps) in performance. Again, a classification of PD should only be given if such inconsistencies and short-term performance decrements are not better explained by interpersonal, intrapersonal, transitional, developmental, or clinical issues.

Interventions for PD will require some form of performance enhancement strategy, which will typically be educational and strategic in nature. Psychological treatment would not be necessary.

It is important to repeat that there must be an absence of transitional, clinical, interpersonal, intrapersonal, and developmental factors to receive a classification of PD. It is therefore critical that the consultant accurately assess the performer's need *prior* to initiating an intervention. We stress this point because, like many clients, some performers may not immediately mention these concerns to the consultant. In fact, consultants who engage in unstructured interviews or assume that the client would certainly note greater concerns if they were present may find out 3 weeks later that the client has more concerns than were originally stated. As such, the consultant cannot automatically assume these issues do not exist, resist asking the important questions, or wait for the client to mention greater concerns. A consultant who focuses exclusively on the performer's stated goals may miss critical psychological concerns, thus making efforts at performance enhancement less successful. Of even greater concern, failure to see subclinical or clinical issues increases the client's personal risk and places the consultant at risk for malpractice.

Performance Dysfunction

The performance dysfunction classification represents issues brought to the performance consultant in which:

- There is a desire to improve performance as either the primary or secondary goal of intervention.
- Past performance has been consistently greater than one's current level of performance, or performance progress is slowed or delayed.
- While the performer is generally psychologically healthy, there are psychological barriers such as transitional, interpersonal, developmental, or schematic issues (intrapersonal, personality, enduring behavioral characteristics) that are negatively affecting the performer.
- Overall psychological and behavioral functioning are either chronically or situationally reduced to a degree.
- Intervention decisions should clearly target the psychological processes underlying the client's performance and nonperformance functioning.

The performance dysfunction classification has two subtypes: Pdy-I and Pdy-II. Pdy-I includes clients whose transitional, interpersonal, developmental, or external life events have led to psychological reactions and have resulted in dysfunctional performance. In contrast, for the Pdy-II client, performance cues and the competitive environment have triggered underlying internal psychological factors such as maladaptive schemas and/or enduring behavioral characteristics such as excessive fear of failure, extreme perfectionism, low frustration tolerance, and irrational need for approval. These schemas and/or personality-based behavioral patterns have subsequently led to performance dysfunction.

While Pdy clients have one or more personal issues in need of remediation, most Pdy clients *initially* seek consultation due to performance
difficulties. The primary complaint or consultation request may appear
to have little to do with the transitional, developmental, interpersonal,
or intrapersonal issues underlying the performance decrements, because
these performers are still generally psychologically healthy and have performed at higher levels in the past. However, subclinical psychological
issues are now impacting the performer in one of two ways. For Pdy-I
clients, transitional issues, current life circumstances, developmental issues, or interpersonal/intrapersonal psychological barriers have resulted
in affective, physiological, or behavioral consequences that impact not
only their ability to reach optimal levels of performance, but also their
ability to navigate some of life's general demands. Pdy-II clients have
underlying cognitive schemas, dispositional personality variables, and
enduring behavioral characteristics that are typically not disruptive. Yet
these traits and characteristics certainly can be exacerbated by increased
life stress. When this occurs, these endogenous psychological factors can
result in some form of dysfunction (such as work, academic, athletic, or
familial/social dysfunction). When working with clients who receive a
Pdy classification, the consultant is encouraged to not overly focus on the
performance issues that the client initially presents. Instead, we suggest
that the consultant carefully assess the performer's schemas, enduring
behavioral characteristics, and current emotional and behavioral functioning, which includes an assessment of the interpersonal/intrapersonal,
work/educational, and recreational domains.

Reports and findings by Meyers, Whelan, and Murphy (1996), Bond
(2001), and Bauman (2000) confirm that Pdy types of cases are frequent
in the day-to-day practice of sport and performance psychology. Although
these professionals did not use the MCS-SP classification system (it had
yet to be developed), they did find that a significant number of athlete
clients who originally sought consultation for performance enhancement
(thus classified as PD) were, after thorough assessment, actually cases
in which performance decrements were primarily due to the clients' interpersonal, intrapersonal, or developmental circumstances (which we
classify as Pdy).

The criteria for Pdy classifications clearly indicate that transitional,
developmental, interpersonal, and intrapersonal issues are the essential
foci of intervention. Such individuals do not have to have a long history
of subclinical barriers to receive a Pdy classification. For the most part,
these are not individuals requiring significant clinical attention. In fact,
Pdy also includes cases in which performers experience persistent though
possibly short-term performance decrements (also known as slumps) that
are *primarily* explained by transitional, developmental, interpersonal, or

intrapersonal factors. A hallmark of Pdy is that personal issues such as these are largely responsible for the performance decrements, and typically also affect the performer's overall psychological functioning and quality of life. As such, these issues are viewed as more significant than performance issues to the performer's overall well-being and adjustment. Common examples of Pdy issues include career/sport transitions, significant family/relationship disruption, death and loss, psychological reactions to non–career-threatening injury, and significant role changes. Also included would be intrapersonal and interpersonal issues such as avoidance, performance anxiety and minor behavioral dysregulation during performance, patterns of overinvolvement or underinvolvement at work, low frustration tolerance, perfectionism, acute stress reactions not meeting the criteria for posttraumatic stress disorder, fear of failure and success, and poor performance-related interpersonal relationships (Gardner & Moore, 2006). The nature of Pdy cases suggests that the consultant's fundamental goal is to foster improvement in both performance *and* psychosocial functioning.

As outlined in chapters 4 through 10, the MAC protocol is specifically designed to be used in a flexible manner with both PD or Pdy clients. The next two classifications—performance impairment and performance termination—are briefly described below. However, the MAC program was not designed for use with clients experiencing PI and PT difficulties. Interested readers are referred to Gardner and Moore (2006) for a comprehensive review of the empirically supported treatments for clients who are experiencing these types of difficulties.

Performance Impairment

The performance impairment classification represents issues brought to the performance consultant in which:

- Diagnosable clinical issues are present that are causing extreme emotional distress and/or behavioral dysregulation, potentially resulting in reduced performance or a complete inability to perform due to outside involvement (league suspension, corporate action, judicial involvement).
- Clinical issues are severely impairing at least one major domain of life (usually more), including social-interpersonal, familial, recreational, self-care, educational, and occupational domains.
- Performance enhancement techniques (including the MAC) may be desired by the client, but are clearly of secondary importance to the significant clinical issues impacting the performer.

- Due to the significance of the clinical issues, it is highly unlikely that developing or refining psychological skills will substantially affect performance issues or the performer's overall psychosocial functioning.

There are two subtypes within the PI classification: PI-I and PI-II. The PI-I designation is given to clients for whom clinical disorders such as affective, eating, anxiety, and posttraumatic stress disorders severely impair overall life functioning and either nearly or completely disable the client's performance. Quite differently, the PI-II designation is given to clients for whom behavioral dysregulation such as drug and alcohol abuse, anger and impulse control disorders, and personality disorders significantly impair one or more major life domains (such as family and work), which may also result in an external decision to limit the performer's participation in his or her given domain. While not required, external limitations may include job suspension or dismissal, judicial actions, legal suspension, and incarceration.

The overall PI classification subsumes issues that can be given formal psychiatric diagnoses according to the *Diagnostic and Statistical Manual of Mental Disorders* (American Psychiatric Association, 2000), and typically includes performers with clear, clinical levels of emotional distress or behavioral difficulty. Although performers experiencing PI will likely report (at least intermittently) significant difficulties with their work/competitive performance, the performance decrements are of secondary importance to the psychological distress and reduced functioning common to these cases. Most of the performance decrements directly result from the psychological distress or behavioral dysregulation the client experiences.

Performance Termination

The performance termination classification represents issues brought to the performance consultant in which:

- The client's primary concerns are related to the multiple stressors and difficulties associated with voluntary or involuntary career completion, where there is little realistic potential for reinstituting or preserving the career.
- Psychological reactions reflecting either a normative or exceptional grieving process (such as anger, depression, and anxiety) may exist, and family and interpersonal issues are likely to warrant significant attention.
- Career realities contraindicate efforts at performance enhancement.

- Counseling or psychological treatment is clearly the intervention of choice, and referrals may be necessary for adjunctive career counseling and financial planning.

Like the other MCS-SP classifications, the performance termination category is comprised of two subtypes: PT-I and PT-II. PT-I applies to cases in which the client's career has ended expectedly (possibly voluntarily) due to any number of possible factors. Most clients will react in a way that is somewhat similar to the normative grieving following the expected death of a loved one. This reaction may include a slow, subclinical progression through the linear stages of shock, denial, anger, depression, and acceptance (Hopson & Adams, 1977; Kubler-Ross, 1969).

PT-II clients typically have a much different reaction, because their careers end unexpectedly and involuntarily. In these cases, the client typically has few, if any, alternative options to maintain the performance career. In addition to facing unexpected career termination, there is also now the need to plan for a new lifestyle and career. The client may experience a severe psychological reaction similar to those who experience a delayed or extreme grief reaction, acute stress reaction, or posttraumatic stress disorder. PT-II clients also tend to progress through the stages of shock, denial, anger, depression, and acceptance (Hopson & Adams, 1977; Kubler-Ross, 1969), but this progression is typically significantly more severe than the experience of PT-I clients. For this reason, PT-II clients usually require greater treatment intensity.

CONCLUSION

Prior to initiating the MAC program, the consultant should have already collected the information necessary for understanding the client's presenting problem in a complete psychosocial context. The goal is an understanding of the relationship between the presenting problem and the vast array of individual client variables. The case formulation method presented here allows for a comprehensive understanding of the client, and an appropriate MCS-SP classification that subsequently either guides the proper delivery of the MAC program or leads to the determination that the performer's needs are beyond the scope of the MAC program (thereby requiring a different type of psychological intervention). This case formulation approach requires that the consultant remain committed to the careful collection of all necessary information and to integrating and synthesizing this information into a sound working model for understanding the performer who is seeking professional services.

Having provided a foundation of a model for understanding functional and dysfunctional performance; the theoretical and empirical evolution of the MAC program; and a comprehensive method of assessment, case formulation, and classification, we proceed with a journey through the MAC program.

PART II

Strategies and Techniques of the MAC Approach to Performance Enhancement

CHAPTER 4

MAC Module 1: Preparing the Client With Psychoeducation

As with all structured psychological interventions, particularly those developed out of the cognitive-behavioral tradition, the first session of the MAC intervention is psychoeducational in nature. Findings in the professional literature suggest that psychological interventions work best when the following three conditions are achieved at the outset of psychological intervention efforts (Castonguay & Beutler, 2006):

1. An effective working alliance between consultant and client.
2. The client gaining a means of reconceptualizing his or her issues or problems into a better explanatory system.
3. Enhanced hope.

With the development of these conditions in mind, the consultant sets the stage for effective intervention by providing an appropriate rationale for the MAC intervention, establishing the foundational purpose and goals of MAC, and building hope and a positive expectancy by demonstrating how the client's performance experiences—both positive and negative—make sense and can be understood from the MAC perspective.

In addition, the rationale for the MAC approach allows the client to quickly understand the difference between MAC and other attempts at performance enhancement that he or she may have experienced, heard about, or assumed and promotes the realization that this training program will require a personal commitment of time and effort. The analogy of building muscle and physical fitness through active effort and regular and consistent work is freely and liberally employed to convey the commitment required to enhance performance by enhancing mental strength.

It is expected that the consultant will have a thorough understanding of functional and dysfunctional human performance, as described in chapter 1, and a comprehensive understanding of the theoretical and empirical basis of MAC, as described in chapter 2. From this knowledge base, the consultant can help clients feel comfortable with the journey on which they are about to embark and understand their positive and negative performance experiences to date. Elite performers tend to be highly suspicious of people outside of their specialty area claiming to have the secret to enhancing performance. In many respects, they are correct. As discussed in chapter 2, in the past, some sport and performance psychologists have used techniques with questionable efficacy. It is imperative that the consultant take the position that the client is the expert in his or her performance domain, and the job of the consultant using the MAC approach is to offer the development of mental skills that, if applied regularly and correctly, can help the elite performer maximize his or her consistency and level of performance through enhanced attention and poise. Consultants who can effectively communicate that it is the *performer* who must make sense of, and determine how to effectively utilize, the MAC skills in one's day-to-day functioning are more likely to be successful.

The following outline summarizes the components of Module 1. Following the presentation of these concepts, the chapter will discuss the common obstacles faced during this critical module and will address considerations for working with clients experiencing performance dysfunction.

Outline of Module 1

1. Introduction
2. Present the Theoretical Rationale for the MAC Program
3. Connect the Rationale to the Client's Personal Performance Experience
4. Explain Automated Self-Regulation of Elite Performance
5. Define Specific Goals of the MAC Training Program
6. Introduce the Brief Centering Exercise

INTRODUCTION

This initial period is devoted to basic introductions, policies, and procedures. During this segment, meeting times and schedules are presented, issues of confidentiality (and its limits) are described, audio- and videotaping procedures (if relevant) are discussed, and issues relating to contacting the consultant between sessions are described. When working in any athletic, business, military, or other organizational system, special care must be taken to address the following topics: (1) how the client has come to this program, (2) who is and is not aware that the client is participating in the program, (3) who is and is not allowed to know about information discussed within sessions, and (4) who is and is not allowed to receive information (and what type) at the conclusion of the program. It cannot be assumed that all clients enter MAC training completely based on their own desire. Coaches, supervisors, and other personnel in management or leadership roles may have requested or insisted upon completion of the program. As such, circumstances of entry into the MAC program need to be fully understood and efforts should be made to develop a collaborative relationship even in such circumstances. In addition, it is critical that an appropriate informed consent be prepared and signed by all clients prior to beginning MAC training.

A more detailed description of these issues is beyond the scope of this text. For a comprehensive discussion of these issues in the practice of sport and performance psychology, readers are referred to Gardner and Moore (2006) and Moore (2003a), each of which have outlined and discussed these ethical-professional issues in greater detail.

PRESENT THE THEORETICAL RATIONALE FOR THE MAC PROGRAM

In this segment of the first module, the consultant engages in a discussion relating to the general purpose of MAC. In simple language, MAC is described to clients as a psychological intervention with the ultimate goal of performance enhancement through enhanced regulation of attention and poise. *Attention* is defined as the capacity to pay attention to task-relevant information as needed. *Poise* is defined as the ability to act in the service of values and goals despite negative internal states such as thoughts, emotions, and physical sensations that the client may be experiencing. These basic MAC goals are described as being achieved through a sequential process of practitioner-client discussion, in-session exercises, and between-session activities to develop greater moment-to-moment self-awareness and increase tolerance of negative thoughts, emotions, and physical sensations. Unlike other approaches to performance enhancement that attempt to teach the client ways to think and feel better, MAC is described as a means of helping the client maintain attention and poise without any need to reduce, limit, or otherwise control these naturally occurring internal experiences. Rather, the goal of MAC is to develop the ability to allow these naturally occurring experiences to come and go as passing and transitory aspects of the human experience. It is essential that this point be made early in the module and repeated frequently throughout sessions, because it is contrary to other common methods of performance enhancement. In fact, for those clients who have previously been exposed to performance enhancement techniques that attempt cognitive and emotional change and control, the MAC goal of allowing internal experiences to occur naturally may initially be seen as counterintuitive.

In this regard, we have found it helpful to ask clients how successful they have been in eliminating negative thoughts or emotions. When they state that this is usually an unsuccessful endeavor, we may ask them to tell us about a person they know who does not experience negative thoughts, emotions, or physical sensations. To reiterate the point, we frequently ask them to tell us about an individual they respect greatly and describe how this individual has eliminated intense emotions, negative thoughts, or uncomfortable physical sensations. Of course, not one client has eliminated these negative internal experiences, and no individual will come to mind when asked about others. The implication becomes immediately clear. High performing individuals perform well *and* have these difficult internal experiences. This brief exercise is similar to the creative hopelessness activities in the clinical ACT protocol (Hayes, et al., 1999), in which the client is helped to recognize the futility and impossibility of having a life with no pain or discomfort.

Connect the Rationale to the Client's Personal Performance Experience

At this point in the module, it is time to discuss the specific goals and expectations that the client brings to the consulting room. Discuss the client's personal experiences and unique concept of optimal performance and performance difficulties. In essence, the client gives a brief performance history, including best and worst performance moments. The consultant should ensure that the discussion includes practice, training, and preparation, because MAC works not only during direct competitive moments, but—and quite possibly more importantly—through a process of enhancing the effort and focus necessary to practice and train effectively.

It is important that the consultant connect the client's performance beliefs, experiences, and desires to the basic MAC model. This discussion is likely to include concepts that elite performers have come across in their reading and previous experiences with coaches, trainers, or sport-performance psychologists. Such concepts may include "flow," "peak performance," "effortless activity," "ideal performance state," "sport confidence," "being in the zone," or "individual zones of optimal functioning." Although the MAC approach does not use such concepts (because they have taken on pop culture meanings with little or no utility for the professional), it is nevertheless important that the consultant discuss how these concepts are reflected in the basic goals of MAC and how the MAC skill-building approach is more likely than other methods to help the client reach his or her desired goals and values.

It is here that the consultant should incorporate information that was collected from the client in the initial interview and/or psychometric testing, as discussed in chapter 3. Hypotheses made by the consultant regarding the issues to be addressed, including a clear explanation that connects problematic processes and problematic outcomes (as discussed earlier in this text), can and should be presented at this time. This promotes the reconceptualization of one's problems in a more understandable way. This process of reconceptualizing one's issues and problems has been related to positive outcomes in other psychological interventions (Castonguay & Beutler, 2006).

Special care should be given to include a discussion of the difference between self-focused and task-focused attention and the relationship of each to functional and dysfunctional performance. The client should be asked to discuss experiences with self- versus task-focused attention in the context of his or her personal performance history. Below is a brief example of a discussion connecting the relationship between functional and dysfunctional performance and self- versus task-focused attention.

CONSULTANT: Can you think about an example in which you performed below what you were expecting?

CLIENT: Sure. A couple of weeks ago I had an awful game. I missed a couple of practices that week and the coach was on me big time.

CONSULTANT: Do you remember what your mind was telling you during the game?

CLIENT: Yeah. . . . I kept wondering if I was running the play right . . . if I was in the right place on the floor.

CONSULTANT: Tell me about another time when you performed closer to your expectation.

CLIENT: (laughs) Actually, that's easy, it was the next game.

CONSULTANT: And what was your mind telling you then?

CLIENT: Hmmm. I don't know that I was thinking about anything. I was in the flow of the game. It seemed so easy. I just played. I reacted to the other team, did what I had to do, and had a great game.

An interaction such as this is then used to illustrate the relationship between self-focused attention and task-focused attention. The emphasis on the self can be seen in the phrases about "wondering if I was running the play right . . . if I was in the right place." On the other hand, this perspective opposes those situations in which the client is focused on the task, which can be seen in the statement, "I reacted to the other team, did what I had to do." Eliciting this type of information is relatively easy and is predictably followed by an expression of awareness on the client's face. We often describe this as the light bulb turning on for the client.

If the client has a difficult time grasping the concept, and cannot offer personal examples, an example of the relationship between focus of attention and sexual performance could be discussed. It will be obvious to nearly every adult that a focus on "How am I doing?" in the context of sexual performance is likely to culminate in less-than-satisfactory performance. Similarly, the experience of being fully engaged in the moment with complete focus on the activities and sensations will almost certainly result in a far different outcome.

At the conclusion of this segment of Module 1, the client is generally asked to complete the Performance Rating Form (see Figure 4.1). The information on this form can be used as a source of conversation and a way to monitor client progress throughout the entire MAC protocol. For ongoing progress monitoring, we suggest having the client complete the form at the end of modules 4 and 8, or after any four-session period when progress evaluation seems logical.

EXPLAIN AUTOMATED SELF-REGULATION OF ELITE PERFORMANCE

At this time, the session should effortlessly move to a discussion of the frequent negative impact of trying to exert conscious control over performance instead of allowing the execution of skills to effortlessly occur. In this regard, the contradiction of efforts to think better, feel better, be positive, and avoid negative self-talk is described and discussed. As a hall of fame professional athlete accurately stated to the first author (Gardner), with whom he worked, the goal of the program is "to get [your] head out of [your] body's way." Essentially, the client is told that:

> The primary goal of the MAC program is to allow your skills and abilities to emerge automatically, with your mind being quiet and focused on only the task at hand.

Performance Rating Form

Initials_____ Date_____ Age_____ Occupation_____ Gender_____

Please list performance barriers that have occurred within the last 2 weeks (such as negative thoughts, negative emotions, interpersonal problems, lack of concentration, etc.).

_____

_____

_____

_____

0	1	2	3	4	5	6	7	8
None		Mild		Moderate		Strong		Extreme

Please rate each of the following using the 0–8 scale above.

Performance Domain	Satisfaction With Performance	Impact of Performance Barrier
Practice/Training		
Competition/Work		
Relationships With Staff		
Relationships With Coworkers/Teammates		
Other (please describe): _____ _____ _____ _____	_____ _____ _____ _____	_____ _____ _____ _____

FIGURE 4.1   Performance Rating Form

It is important to stress that a fundamental goal of MAC is to remove the effects of excessive cognitive activity from performance. At this step, it is often helpful to discuss how efforts to *control* thoughts and emotions or efforts to *act* on thoughts and emotions can distract from and thus hinder ideal performance. Clients will typically be able to provide examples of this from their own experience. The consultant should once again ask how well efforts to control thoughts and emotions have worked for them in the past, and what specific efforts they have utilized. For most clients, the recognition that these internal events do not have to be eliminated or controlled is a freeing experience. Clients frequently enter the program with the belief that eliminating or controlling internal states is possible and helpful, yet believe that because they have been unsuccessful at achieving this goal, they are somehow defective or unskilled. When clients realize the impossibility of truly eliminating or controlling these internal processes, they can then become fully engaged and excited about the program to come.

DEFINE SPECIFIC GOALS OF THE MAC TRAINING PROGRAM

In this final segment of Module 1, the discussion should clearly restate the importance of enhanced attention to performance-relevant internal and external cues and enhanced poise in response to the obstacles, challenges, and unexpected events inherent in any elite area of human performance. Although it may seem that this topic has been covered already, it is important to discuss these goals often. The consultant should always recognize that he or she only *indirectly* enhances the client's performance. Performance is improved by learning to practice and train more efficiently and consistently and from the enhancement of psychological skills such as task-focused attention and poise.

The consultant can use this opportunity to present the distinction between control (as promoted by traditional performance enhancement efforts) and the concept of acceptance that is a core MAC feature. Previous to trying the MAC approach, clients have often been told repeatedly that if they only could feel less bad, have fewer negative thoughts, were more confident, or were able to relax and put themselves in "the zone," they would excel in their chosen field. Instead, the MAC consultant suggests the questions: What if all of the effort put into thinking and feeling a certain way was doomed to fail? What if no one could consistently control his or her feelings, and what if it was not even necessary to do so? What would the person then do? The purpose of this series of questions is to help the client consider an alternative to the control agenda. This discussion, with relevant connections to the client's own experiences, inevitably leads to the central conclusion of MAC and all acceptance-based psychological interventions:

> The struggle to be without distress is the problem, not the presence of these thoughts and feelings.

Thus, once again, we highlight for the client that the concept of needing to think and feel good in order to perform optimally should be replaced with the concept of developing the ability to feel or think badly *and* perform optimally.

It is here that the consultant introduces and describes the training of mindfulness (presented in chapter 2), including the importance of the regular use of mindfulness exercises. As part of this introduction, and central to the purpose of integrating mindfulness into the MAC, the concept of mindful awareness is presented. *Mindful awareness* is the process by which one learns to notice and accept a variety of thoughts and emotions as naturally occurring phenomena that are not necessary to control. Similarly, the concept of mindful attention is presented. *Mindful attention* is defined as the ability to self-regulate task attention. In essence, the client is presented with the idea (frequently repeated throughout the program) that a basic goal of MAC is to change statements such as, "I want to perform well *but* I am thinking negatively or feeling badly," to "I want to perform well *and* I am thinking negatively or feeling badly." It is pointed out that, within the first phrase, the initial segment does not allow the second segment to coexist, while the second phrase allows room for both segments to happen simultaneously.

Of course, the consultant must ensure that the client is aware that, as a skill-building approach, there will be regular between-session assignments and exercises to be completed. We highly suggest not describing this as *homework*. The tendency during cognitive-behavioral interventions is to refer to between-session exercises as *homework;* for many individuals, this term stimulates a natural aversion and avoidance response left over from the school years. Few children enjoy the concept of or time spent completing homework, and even fewer adults would like to feel as though they are children back in school. *Exercises,* or between-session assignments, on the other hand, are accepted as part of training programs of all types. At this time, the consultant may choose to once again make a comparison to working out, in which increased strength does not simply come from entering a gym, but instead comes from regularly extending the workload and pushing oneself to higher and higher limits. This will be understood by elite performers in every field, and the use of this analogy will effectively communicate the requirement for consistent client effort in the service of his or her own personal growth and development.

INTRODUCE THE BRIEF CENTERING EXERCISE

Finally, as a way of demonstrating the experiential aspect of this program, and as a way of initiating a focus on training mindful attention, the session ends with a brief mindfulness exercise known as the Brief Centering Exercise, shown in Figure 4.2 (Eifert & Forsyth, 2005).

The form entitled What I Have Learned About Performance and Myself (see Figure 4.3) should be given to the client at the completion of each session (especially after the first three or four sessions). The client should be instructed to complete the form as soon as possible after the session. This form is intended to allow the client to see that he or she is, in fact, increasing knowledge and self-awareness. In addition, despite regular smiles and gestures of agreement and understanding within sessions, this form allows the consultant to monitor gaps in development.

At the end of the first session, we also suggest that you provide a copy of the handout Preparing for MAC (see Figure 4.4), which provides the client with an overview of basic essentials for beginning this—or any—psychological intervention.

COMMON PROBLEMS SEEN IN MODULE 1

The following are common problems that we have noticed with our clients and when supervising consultants new to the MAC performance enhancement training program.

Lack of a Thorough and Comprehensive Understanding of Basic MAC Principles

We cannot stress enough the need for consultants working with elite performers for the purpose of performance enhancement to understand the fundamental principles underlying functional and dysfunctional performance, as well as the fundamental principles of MAC. This is especially true for those who have worked in sport-performance psychology or in clinical-counseling psychology, because many such practitioners have been trained in change-based procedures. For such consultants, the idea

Brief Centering Exercise

This brief exercise will help you focus on the immediate moment. You will also begin the process of developing the skill of mindful attention. This exercise should take you about 5 minutes to complete. As with any other exercise or activity, before you start, remember that success requires the development of specific skills, and a commitment to working on the development of these skills is the first step to success.

Please find a comfortable sitting position. Notice the position of your feet, arms, and hands. Allow your eyes to close gently. [pause 10 seconds] Breathe in and out gently and deeply several times. Notice the sound and feel of your own breath as you breathe in and out. [pause 10 seconds]

At this time, focus your attention on your surroundings. Notice any sounds that may be occurring. What sounds are occurring inside the room? What sounds are occurring outside the room? [pause 10 seconds] Now focus your attention on the areas where your body touches the chair in which you are sitting. Notice the physical sensations that occur from this contact. [pause 10 seconds] Now notice the spot where your hands are touching the front of your legs. [pause 10 seconds] Now notice any sensations that may be occurring in the rest of your body and notice how they may change over time without any effort on your part. [pause 10 seconds] Don't try to alter these sensations; just notice them as they occur. [pause 10 seconds]

Now, let your thoughts focus on why you have chosen to pursue this program. [pause 10 seconds] See if you can notice any doubts or other thoughts without doing anything but noticing them. Just notice your reservations, concerns, and worries as though they are elements of a parade passing through your mind. [pause 10 seconds] See if you can simply notice them and acknowledge their presence. [pause 10 seconds] Don't try to make them go away or change them in any way. [pause 10 seconds] Now allow yourself to focus on what you want your performance life to be about. What is most important to you? What do you want to do with your skills? [pause 10 seconds]

Remain comfortable for a few more moments and slowly let yourself focus once again on any sounds and movements occurring around you. [pause 10 seconds] Once again notice your own breathing. [pause 10 seconds] When you are ready, open your eyes and notice that you feel focused and attentive.

FIGURE 4.2   Brief Centering Exercise

What I Have Learned About Performance and Myself

Initials_____ Date_____ Age_____ Occupation_____ Gender_____

During each session, and across each week of the MAC training program, you are likely to learn a variety of new things about yourself and human performance. After you leave each week's session, I would like you to complete this form as soon as possible. The purpose of this is to ensure that you are learning and remembering the important concepts from each of our sessions together. This allows me to make sure that you are developing all the necessary performance enhancement skills included in the MAC program.

1._____

_____

_____

_____

2._____

_____

_____

_____

3._____

_____

_____

_____

4._____

_____

_____

_____

5._____

_____

_____

FIGURE 4.3   What I Have Learned About Performance and Myself

Now that you have learned about human performance and the MAC training program for performance enhancement, it is time to prepare yourself for our work together. Changing the way we respond to what our mind tells us (our thoughts) and what we feel (our emotions and physical sensations) is not easy, but not impossible either. You have already achieved things that others told you were not possible. As you know, it helps to approach developing new skills with the correct attitude and mind-set. Here are some tips to keep in mind as you begin the journey of mental skill development, the MAC way.

- Developing the mental skills of mindful attention, mindful awareness, and poise requires an active effort and commitment, both in our sessions and between our sessions. Think of this as equivalent to physical training or physical rehabilitation. In many respects, the saying, "no pain, no gain" is appropriate to what you are about to undertake.

- Remain curious and keep an open mind about what you hear and what you are being asked to do. Many of the concepts are different from what you have been taught to believe. See the MAC program as an opportunity to experiment and learn something new.

- To increase the likelihood of success, keep your expectations reasonable and choose areas to work on that are manageable and realistic.

- Accept the idea that enhancing your performance is an evolutionary process and not a single revolutionary event.

- Don't be overly hard on yourself for slips, errors, or inconsistent success with the program. Your skills will develop in the same way that all previous skills have developed in your life—with hard work, repeated practice, and gradually over time.

- Most importantly, remember that your presence here is not because you have failed or because there is something wrong with you. The attitude, "just do it," is not enough... if it was, everyone would be an elite performer!

FIGURE 4.4   Preparing for MAC

that changing one's thoughts and emotions is not necessary for enhanced human functioning is as foreign as it is to the clients we serve. We cannot state strongly enough that consultants who cannot understand, accept, and essentially buy in to the concept of mindful acceptance and commitment to valued directions are probably not ready to utilize this program. The reason is very simple: they are likely to send confusing and counterproductive mixed messages in the intervention strategies and goals.

An example of this comes from a recent session completed by a MAC trainee. Toward the end of an otherwise exceptional first session, and immediately following the presentation of the Brief Centering Exercise, the student remarked, "This will really help you if you do it when you feel yourself getting upset. You will feel so much better." Of course, the problem here is that MAC does *not* have as its goal the reduction of negative affect. While at times this may seem helpful and ultimately can be seen as a reasonable long-term secondary benefit of mindfulness and acceptance-based procedures, it is absolutely contrary to the fundamental goal of MAC, which is that negative thoughts and emotions are absolute realities that cannot, and need not, be eliminated or controlled. As such, the message of "do x or y and you will feel better," presents a mixed message and places the client in a confusing situation in which the overlearned automatic desire to feel better is likely to predominate. Upon discussion with the student, it became clear that this unintentional error was in fact representative of his own personal ambivalence regarding the basic foundation of MAC.

Of course, this is not to say that even the most fervent supporters of this approach will not on occasion be prone to the culturally accepted idea that thinking better and feeling better are critical to functioning (performing) better. All those engaged in using and teaching MAC must be ever mindful of the societal influences that reinforce this notion, from parenting skills that exaggerate the need for children to feel better at the moment (rather than functioning better in the future), to pharmaceutical ad campaigns that suggest that, through the use of the correct medication, you will feel better, always smile, and automatically live a happier and more productive life. The desire for a quick fix can be seen in many circles, including through the increasing use of performance-enhancing substances by athletes.

It is generally accepted by those who have adopted the "third wave" of behavioral psychology that living one's life engaged in the personal practice of mindfulness and acceptance is necessary for effective professional service delivery. We suggest conveying to your client that you are both fallible humans and that you too have to work on—and at times even struggle—with being mindful, accepting, and committed. This stated recognition that both the client and consultant are in life together, with all the inevitable struggles that this entails, will go a long way in allowing you to effectively relate to and serve your client in a collaborative manner throughout the MAC program.

The Use of Overly Complicated Language (Jargon)

The use of jargon, or overly complicated professional language (often referred to within psychology as *psychobabble*), is a problem sometimes encountered with intellectually gifted individuals who are so immersed in their field that they lose sight of the impact that this use of language has on their clients. While the use of jargon has negative consequences when it occurs with clinical or counseling clients, it is even more problematic in performance settings in which the elite performer does not want to see the consultant as someone who cannot relate or who has no personal humanity. In fact, the overuse of jargon in the first session may result in premature termination from the program. The use of overly intellectual terminology pushes away the client rather than bringing him or her closer into a collaborative working relationship. It conveys distance, not warmth, and suggests an arrogant mentality rather than a real human connection. Elite performers who we have worked with over the years have often commented (well after the fact) about our ease of communicating in everyday language, which has been reported to us as portraying true confidence and professionalism.

The following example of the overuse of jargon comes from a session tape of a consultant in her first session with a high-level salesperson. She is attempting to convey the basic goals of the MAC program.

CONSULTANT: So, I want you to fully understand that optimal performance is based on the ability to maintain performance-appropriate task-focused attention so as to not allow for problems in the discrepancy adjustment portion of self-regulation. And so, we will use mindfulness meditation to decrease self-focused attention through enhanced mindful attention and awareness and promote automatic task-focused attention. Is that clear?

CLIENT: Not really.

CONSULTANT: Which part didn't you get?

CLIENT: (Laughing) Well, I remember your name.

In this brief interaction, it is obvious that the consultant did not translate the information into more useable language that could promote active discussion. Something that we repeatedly stress to students is the need for all helping professions (particularly those working with elite performers) to present their knowledge within the context of their own personalities and in a language and manner to which the client can easily relate. If you find yourself talking to your clients in a way that is different than the way you would explain MAC to your friends or family members, you are probably not approaching it well. Becoming personally mindful of your manner of interacting with clients is as critical when working with elite performers as it is when working with clients experiencing more severe clinical difficulties.

Not Accepting Acceptance

Some clients have a particularly difficult time moving from change-based to acceptance-based ideas. This is likely to be the most common obstacle for the successful completion of the first MAC module. In some cases, the client will openly and directly challenge the idea that people can perform better, even optimally, without having to control or limit the types of thoughts or emotions they experience. Remember, this concept is contrary to the reinforced notion of Western society suggesting just the opposite. As noted in chapter 2, only recently have more Eastern concepts relating to acceptance been integrated into psychological science. Letting go of control notions and accepting acceptance will not come easy for some. In response to this, it is helpful for the consultant to validate the client's struggle to view these concepts differently. We also recommend that, rather than arguing or debating with the client over this issue, the consultant should suggest that the client *consider* the acceptance alternative and gently ask the client to consider which model provides a better fit for the reality of life and human performance. The first author (Gardner) often tells clients that, when they can identify a performer in their specialty who has truly been able to eliminate or control (not just respond better to) all troubling thoughts or emotions (at all times and in all ways), he will reconsider his position.

The issue of accepting the acceptance model becomes even more difficult when working with reactant or disagreeable/resistant clients (see chapter 3). The professional literature has discussed how these individuals respond best to a more nondirective approach. Thus, the less the consultant pushes the client and instead allows the client to come to this new place in his or her own time, the more likely it is that intervention success will be attained. The assessment of reactance is suggested in the case formulation method (see chapter 3), and, as such, reactant clients will typically be recognized prior to beginning the MAC program.

The Uncommitted Client Who Has Been Cajoled Into the MAC Program

The issue of the cajoled client arises in both clinical and performance-enhancement practice. Some clients may have been overtly or subtly coerced by family, coach, management, staff, or teammates/coworkers to seek out sport or performance psychology as a means of enhancing their performance. These individuals usually come reluctantly, or at least with a great deal of ambivalence. This is especially true for those whose sport or cultural background equates anything psychological to weakness and personal problems. In such cases, the consultant should patiently help the client understand and agree with the need for performance enhancement efforts and come to personally believe that enhanced performance is in their own best interest (regardless of the referral source).

Some professionals suggest that avoiding the use of such words as *psychology, psychologist, mental,* or any derivation thereof would easily rectify this situation. In fact, however, the experience of the authors suggests that it is not words or titles that matter, but rather the attitude and behavior of the consultant. If you believe in what you do, then show it, explain why you feel as you do, and convey the down-to-earth confidence that inspires others to believe in you. Although easy to say, we recognize that this is not always easy to do, especially for the novice professional.

The Client Has Had Negative Previous Experiences With Psychology and/or Performance Enhancement

Similar to the uncommitted client, the client who has had negative prior experience with psychology or performance enhancement efforts will potentially be skeptical, and may possibly overtly challenge the ideas presented by the consultant. We suggest that the consultant respond to this type of client in much the same way as he or she would respond to an uncommitted client. The difference is that the consultant will need to validate the concerns and negative reactions of the client by professing full agreement with the client regarding his or her earlier experiences. Performance-enhancement services are often oversold, and many have little likelihood of true success. Thus, it is likely that the reasons these earlier experiences did not work the way the client had expected was because they were insufficient techniques to achieve the client's goals. We have sided with our clients numerous times, suggesting that such experiences were exactly the reason for the development of the MAC approach. We then state that, although it is completely understandable that they would be skeptical, we would like them to suspend their skepticism and give this very different approach a chance.

Although this approach is likely to be effective, one possible complication is when the reason for the previous negative experience was not the technique or strategy used, but rather some aspect of the consultant personality, style, or behavior. In this situation, we suggest simply posing the question, "If you had a physician who behaved that way or did those things, would you swear off the practice of medicine or would you seek out a more competent professional with whom you felt comfortable and trusted?" This approach, although not guaranteed to work, at least conveys a validation of their problem while presenting your belief that the conclusion he or she is reaching may not be rational or in the client's best interest.

MODULE 1 CONSIDERATIONS FOR WORKING WITH CLIENTS EXPERIENCING PERFORMANCE DYSFUNCTION

As noted, a significant issue in the field of performance psychology has been the tendency to view all clients desiring performance enhancement as free of psychological difficulties (often referred to as barriers). The unfortunate binary view that clients are either psychologically healthy or have clinical disorders has hindered the growth of the field and has, as our research described earlier suggests, resulted in a subset of clients who do not receive the appropriate interventions to meet their specific needs. Readers interested in a more comprehensive discussion of this issue are referred to Gardner and Moore (2006).

Given the importance of this issue, clients who have been identified as experiencing performance dysfunction during the assessment process described in chapter 3 require modifications of the MAC protocol to address the specific processes related to their dysfunction. In each subsequent session, additions or modifications to the basic MAC protocol must be undertaken. It also should be pointed out that, in such cases, it is likely that the seven-session format would need to be modified to ensure that the problematic processes are fully addressed. The modifications will typically include incorporating techniques and strategies usually found in more comprehensive clinical acceptance-based protocols, but will be integrated within the overall MAC context.

In this first module, the modification consists of simply adding a discussion of the client's performance dysfunction and its associated processes. This would be done during the third segment of Module 1 when the MAC rationale is connected to the client's personal performance history and experience. The following vignette provides an example of this process:

CONSULTANT: Now that I have given you an overview of our model and how this program will work, why don't you tell me how you see this fitting into the issues we discussed earlier as part of our initial assessment?

CLIENT: Well, like we talked about, I seem to be going backward. I am learning more about sales presentations, and I have received a lot of training and good experiences, but my performance in these situations is getting worse and worse. From our discussion, I can see that my attention has certainly become more focused on myself, how I look, how I sound . . . to the point that I even forget what I am in the middle of saying! I am so not connected to the people around me, and the presentation that I have prepared for, that it is frightening. I spend so much more time thinking and worrying about my work, and the implications for and about me, that I am doing worse and worse, and enjoying it less and less.

CONSULTANT: Let me connect what you are telling me to some of the information we collected in the assessment we recently completed together. According to some of the questionnaires you completed, your level of worry is near levels seen in people with an anxiety disorder. Now, you do not meet criteria for such a problem, and don't have the symptoms typically seen in anxiety disorders, and you don't have the general life disruption that occurs with disorders of this type. But the level of worry that you seem to experience, as you yourself have described, and as we can measure, suggests an issue that we should address during the MAC program. In the course of developing new skills, we will also attempt to reduce the impact that worry has on your performance. Remember, our goal will not necessarily be to reduce or eliminate these thoughts, but have you view them differently so that they become less disruptive to you.

CLIENT: Okay, that seems to make sense. I would really like to stop fighting myself so much.

In this short interaction, the consultant connected the problem to the assessment data and connected both the problem and the data to the model. In addition, this issue has been added as an additional goal of the MAC program for this client. The consultant also clearly presented that they would work on changing the *relationship* that the client has with worry, and not necessarily a *reduction* in the amount of worry.

There are many possible psychological barriers to performance that do not reach clinical levels. The practitioner should avoid the tendency to ignore or avoid these issues because the client simply desires performance enhancement; and, likewise, the consultant should not overpathologize clients by diagnosing clinical disorders that do not exist and subsequently beginning full psychological treatment when intensive interventions are not indicated.

CHAPTER 5

MAC Module 2: Introducing Mindfulness and Cognitive Defusion

The primary intent of MAC Module 2 is an expanded introduction to the importance of mindful awareness and mindful attention in promoting behavior change in general and enhanced performance in particular. In addition, it is during this module that cognitive defusion (the ability to view what the mind tells us as separate and different from literal truth) is introduced and discussed.

During Module 2, the practitioner describes mindfulness as a *process* and points out that mindfulness exercises are a means to develop specific skills of self-regulated attention, cognitive defusion, and personal awareness. It is also important to stress the need for regular daily practice of mindfulness exercises throughout the program and beyond. In this regard, the goal is to help the client to understand the relationship between self-awareness and the context in which new learning can occur. From this perspective, self-awareness allows for overlearned automatic behaviors that do not work to be replaced by more functional new behavior that is in the client's best interest. Over time, it is expected that, as a new way of thinking about one's thoughts (metacognition) and emotions evolves through the use of mindfulness and cognitive defusion, the client will find that his or her behavior will become more functional (in both training *and* competition).

In the early part of Module 2, the consultant should engage the client in a review of the What I Have Learned Form from Module 1. This review should also include some time to respond to reactions or answer questions generated by the previous session.

The session progresses to a discussion of the primary topics of Module 2—self-awareness and mindfulness—and will particularly focus on how these concepts relate to human performance. This discussion includes an introduction to the concept that thoughts (or "things your mind tells you," as we refer to them) are learned internal events that do not always reflect absolute reality and do not necessarily require action. Rather, our thoughts, learned throughout our lives as language associated with particular events, come and go if we just allow them to. Our thoughts can be triggered by a wide variety of visual, auditory, or other stimuli and are learned through association with historical events. The purpose of mindfulness, at least in part, is to develop the ability to notice internal processes nonjudgmentally and then refocus on the performance or task at hand. During this discussion, the consultant helps the client think *about* his or her thoughts, and encourages the client to consider that thoughts are simply passing events that may or may not accurately reflect the realities surrounding the client.

The primary means of promoting self-awareness throughout the MAC program is the during- and between-session use of a variety of mindfulness exercises intended to enhance awareness of internal and external events and enhance the self-regulation of attention (particularly important for optimal performance). As MAC seeks to decrease our view of thoughts as absolute realities, enhance our capacity to view emotions as experiences that do not require reduction or avoidance, and increase the frequency and intensity of values-directed committed behavior, the enhancement of the client's self-awareness is a crucial component of the MAC program.

Outline of Module 2

1. Brief Centering Exercise
2. Discussion of the What I Have Learned Form
3. Check for and Respond to Questions or Uncertainties Regarding the Previous Session
4. Rationale and Importance of Mindfulness
5. Discussion of Between-Session Exercises: What I Have Learned Form, Brief Centering Exercise, and Washing a Dish Mindfulness Exercise
6. Review Session
7. Brief Centering Exercise

BRIEF CENTERING EXERCISE

We suggest that Module 2—and all subsequent modules—begin with the same Brief Centering Exercise that ended the previous session. This allows continued practice and promotes an in-the-moment focus on the current session. Immediately following this brief exercise, the consultant should ask for the client's reactions and normalize the experience that he or she is likely to have during early attempts at mindfulness exercises. Typical of early experiences, clients will describe having a difficult time remaining on task during the exercises and will describe how difficult it was to prevent their thoughts from drifting. It is important that the client develop the capacity to notice and accept distractions and notice boredom or thoughts relating to a desire to be doing something else. Clients are helped to see that having these thoughts are normal and are, in fact, not problematic. In fact, the client is encouraged to have these thoughts, not fight them. The purpose is to engage in the centering exercise *while* having these thoughts, as opposed to viewing the exercise as not doable *because* of the thoughts and end-feelings that may occur. Clients may struggle with the idea that they do not have to control or eliminate thoughts and feelings. As such, this struggle should be validated as normal, and the consultant can explain that this reaction is seen in nearly all clients as they begin the MAC program. The consultant should also point out that struggling with this very new idea is actually *necessary* for the purpose of the MAC program to be truly understood. It is imperative that the client not be left feeling frustrated or defeated. Validating and normalizing these early experiences is critical and, in fact, can be seen as the first step to enhanced self-awareness. We must know where our thoughts naturally go before we can learn to let go and move our attention elsewhere as needed. It also may be beneficial to again relate these concepts and activities to the ultimate goal of enhanced performance.

DISCUSSION OF THE WHAT I HAVE LEARNED FORM

At this point, the consultant will collect the What I Have Learned Form handed out to the client at the end of the last session. If the form has not been completed, it is essential to discuss the reasons. If the incomplete assignment was due to lack of clarity regarding the directions (not typical), some discussion regarding between-session contact with the consultant for the purpose of clarification should occur. Typically, clients fail to complete assignments because they: (1) did not see the purpose, (2) simply chose to not engage in the activity due to a belief that performance enhancement should involve only once-a-week activity on their part, or (3) wanted to avoid the discomfort that may have come from being unable (or believing themselves unable) to adequately record what was discussed in the previous session. This last reason could suggest either a lack of new learning or perfectionistic reluctance to write anything down for fear that it will not be completely correct. Whatever the reason, these issues should be explored. Additional perusal of the case formulation and preintervention assessment data may also offer clues, such as issues of perfectionism or concern about the approval or disapproval of the consultant. Although the consultant should not belabor the point with the client, this is a good opportunity to reiterate that performance enhancement requires more than session attendance. Following this discussion, there is another opportunity to discuss the importance of between-session work and to state that it is not necessary to complete perfect assignments. This issue also can be connected to the concept of professional training (physical, academic, etc.), in which regular and consistent effort is required to learn a skill of any kind.

This issue of not completing assignments or exercises is likely to be seen in all clients, manifesting itself in different frequencies, at different times, and for different reasons throughout the entire MAC program. The following brief vignette is an example of a typical interchange involving this issue.

CONSULTANT: Let's take a look at the What I Have Learned Form that you completed after our session last week.

CLIENT: Well, I really didn't have a chance to do it. Things were pretty hectic last week.

CONSULTANT: I have no doubt you were busy, but do you think if you were getting paid a thousand dollars to do it you might have found time?

CLIENT: (Laughs) Yes, I guess I would have. I sat down to do it, but I got a little anxious because I wasn't sure what I was supposed to write down, so I put it off, and kept finding other things that I had to do instead.

CONSULTANT: Okay. I understand you put it off and felt better right away. There are two things for us to talk about, though. First, let's review the directions to make sure you truly understand what is being asked of you, and then let's take a look at the larger issue of putting off something that is in your best interest in order to feel better in the moment.

CLIENT: I really did understand what I was supposed to do, I just wasn't sure if what I began to think about was correct. I know I have a problem giving all of myself until I am sure it's going to be good enough.

CONSULTANT: Fair enough. Let's talk about how that fits with our description of the MAC program.

In this vignette, the client describes what most practitioners see on a fairly regular basis. These types of issues always must be connected back to the basic MAC model. This enhances the likelihood of future adherence and helps promote the development of both self-awareness and a willingness to experience difficult internal states while remaining committed to values-directed activities. It cannot be stressed too strongly that all client issues relating to performance will at some time and in some way manifest themselves within sessions. The ability to note these in-session manifestations, referred to in the clinical literature as *clinically relevant behaviors* (Kohlenberg & Tsai, 1995) and respond to them as a unique opportunity to promote appropriate client change is the hallmark of an elite consultant in professional psychology. As we suggest to novice MAC consultants:

It is imperative that the consultant utilizing MAC be mindful of client behaviors that reflect the same processes that may negatively impact performance in out-of-session situations.

CHECK FOR AND RESPOND TO QUESTIONS OR UNCERTAINTIES REGARDING THE PREVIOUS SESSION

Logically connected to—and in most cases directly emanating from—the discussion of the What I Have Learned Form, is a brief check for whether the client is having difficulty understanding or has uncertainties regarding the material presented in the previous module. It is important that each MAC session contain an opportunity for questions and uncertainties to be expressed and processed, because the MAC approach is intended to be sequential and cumulative. This discussion will at times be quite rapid, as many clients demonstrate full understanding of the concepts and practices covered to date, or may take somewhat longer if the client poses questions that require the consultant to cover previously described concepts, processes, or rationale. Clients should be reinforced with a great deal of praise and support for their openness and honesty in asking questions. In addition, silence should not necessarily be interpreted as complete understanding of the material, especially if the What I Have Learned Form was either not completed or completed in a cursory manner. Especially early in the MAC protocol, the consultant may want to take a little extra time to check for gaps in client understanding. This will go a long way in promoting successful outcomes with the MAC program.

RATIONALE AND IMPORTANCE OF MINDFULNESS

After making sure no questions or uncertainties remain, the consultant moves on to define and explain the central role of mindfulness in the MAC approach to performance enhancement. It is at this point that the consultant should administer the Mindfulness Attention Awareness Scale (Brown & Ryan, 2003), which provides a convenient and effective measure of mindful attention and mindful awareness. This measure should be given again at the completion of the MAC program (and midway through the MAC program if so desired) to assess changes in necessary mindfulness skills.

The consultant should describe the benefits of being completely immersed "in the moment" of one's performance activity and liberally use examples from the client's personal performance history. An additional benefit of mindful awareness is the enhanced ability to recognize distracters and employ mindful attention to refocus as needed on the task at hand.

It is also important to discuss what mindfulness is *not*. Although mindfulness may promote a sense of calm, mindfulness exercises are not a form of relaxation or positive thinking. It does not seek to promote relaxation, but rather seeks to enhance self-awareness and the subsequent capacity to notice and be free from habitual reactions. In addition, the goal is to pay attention to one's thoughts as objects of attention. Mindfulness is not a trancelike state, nor does it promote a blank mind. In essence, the goal is not to change or leave one's experience, but rather to become more aware (more conscious) of experiences moment-to-moment. We have found, both with ourselves and with numerous clients, that truly accepting this distinction can be difficult at first, especially because the use of mindfulness techniques can lead to a relaxed physical and mental state and can reduce the cognitive noise in one's head. We often ask our clients to describe to us the goal of mindfulness and the associated exercises, because listening to their descriptions can illuminate gaps in their understanding of the constructs.

It is at this point of Module 2 that the consultant first presents the concept of *cognitive fusion*—earlier defined as the process by which an individual views and responds to thoughts as absolute truths that must be responded to in some way. Here, the consultant provides the client with some explanation regarding the (often negative) impact of thinking on performance. Thoughts have meaning because of our ongoing lifelong learning process. There is a learned relationship between the content of a thought and actual historical events that one has experienced. In this regard, thoughts associated with a particular event are often different from the event itself, but we tend to react as though the thoughts *about an event* and the *event itself* are the same. As such, we may respond to our thoughts about some item or event in our lives as though we are responding to the item or event itself.

Cognitive fusion is the treatment of thoughts as though they are what our minds say they are.

For example, the thought, "I am thinking that I can't work for her" is vastly different than the thought, "I can't work for her." In the first statement, the thought is viewed as simply a thought; in the second statement, the thought is perceived as an absolute statement of fact reflecting some higher truth.

Thoughts also take the form of rules, which are linguistic representations of one's learning history. For example, if we have had negative experiences with verbally aggressive authority figures, we may develop strongly held internal rules suggesting something similar to, "If I try to please aggressive people in a position of authority, I will ultimately get put down." This rule, often referred to as a *schema* (Young et al., 2003), then directs our choices and actions. So, when put into a new situation that involves an aggressive boss or coach, rather than responding to the actual situation, we may instead choose actions based on our preconceived rule. As a result, we may act in ways that do not promote the development of an alternative rule or, most importantly, do not lead to actions that make possible personal success and satisfaction.

It is in this segment of Module 2 that we explain to the client the distinction between a reaction to an event (e.g., a coach or boss screams at the client in a public setting and he becomes angry and embarrassed) and thoughts about such events (e.g., when recounting the story to a friend, he becomes angry as he remembers the event). After presenting this concept, it is helpful to elicit an example that has personal relevance to the client to ensure and reinforce learning.

Essentially, you are presenting to your clients the idea that, in the MAC approach, you will help them learn to distinguish between what *is* and what the mind *tells us* it is. At this time, we suggest asking the client to discuss several additional examples from the client's life that reflect this concept. Having the client present several personal examples begins the process of cognitive *de*fusion, which is when the individual can create a distance between content or absolute meaning of words and the relationship or believability of those words. Because this concept can be confusing, asking the client to provide personal examples is also a way of ensuring that he or she fully understand this important concept. The following vignette provides an example of the process of cognitive defusion. The client is a writer who would like to enhance his work performance. The client is able to provide his own example of cognitive defusion.

CONSULTANT: You mentioned to me when we first met that your fiancé has in the past suffered from panic attacks following strenuous exercise and then stopped exercising because of them, so I will use that as an explanation of cognitive fusion. It is likely that, when exercising, your fiancé would naturally experience shallow breathing and a more rapid pulse rate. Now, his mind told him that these sensations might mean that he is having a heart attack and he then responded to the words, thoughts, and images of a heart attack, which would obviously result in an even greater physiological reaction. What became dangerous to your fiancé was not the reality of the increased pulse and other physiological reactions, but rather the associations and reactions he had to the words that his mind was telling himself. Now, the real problem is that the only way he could guarantee not having the reaction was to restrict his activities more and more, and thus work out less and less. Also, his trying to not think about it probably led him to think about it even more. The key is not to change the content of what his mind was telling him, but rather to recognize that his thoughts were simply words that he could notice and allow to pass (as uncomfortable as they might be). And these words did not mean that the things he was imagining were in fact about to happen. In essence, thoughts do not make facts! As another example, you certainly have walked out in the cold and said something like, "damn, I'm going to freeze to death out here!" Now, if you really believed those words, you would certainly have become anxious, but, since you know they were just words you long ago learned to use in such situations, you didn't believe what your mind was telling you and you just ignored the words and went on with your business. Can you think of a similar example of your own thoughts when having trouble writing that would in some way be similar to this process?

CLIENT: Wow, I really can. Yesterday actually, I sat down to work on this project and began thinking, "this is way too hard," "my work shouldn't be that hard," and "I don't think I can do this."

CONSULTANT: And how did you respond to those things that your mind was telling you?

CLIENT: Well, I felt pretty sad, and pretty bad about myself, and decided to watch some TV and start again the next day.

CONSULTANT: So, comparing that to the example I gave about your fiancé, how could you respond differently to what your mind tells you?

CLIENT: Well, I guess I can tell myself I really can do the work.

CONSULTANT: Yeah, I guess you could, but that would still leave you dependent on what your mind tells you. How could you respond differently so that the content of your thoughts doesn't really matter?

CLIENT: Let me think about it for a minute. (pause). Well, I suppose that I can just remind myself that my mind is at it again, and just get down to work regardless of what stuff is going on inside.

CONSULTANT: You got it! They're just words, noise that you have learned over the years. In that example, you are having the thoughts but not buying into the thoughts. The focus has to be on what you are doing and really want to get done.

In the vignette previously presented, the client quickly grasps the concept but, as almost all clients do, will first interpret cognitive defusion as another form of cognitive change. We emphasize that the difference between changing how we *view* our thoughts—sometimes described as the relationship we have with our thoughts—needs to be differentiated from changing the actual content of our thoughts. In essence, the concept of *having* a thought versus *buying into* a thought is differentiated. It is explained to the client that there will be a number of in-session exercises that will help in the process of cognitive defusion. We have found that, instead of using the word *thoughts,* using the phrase *what our mind tells us* or similar variants such as *what our thoughts tell us* makes the point clear in a subtle yet consistent way.

It is at this time that the role of mindfulness training in the process of cognitive defusion is presented. In essence, clients cannot defuse successfully until they have some ability to decenter from what their mind tells them enough to recognize that it is occurring. The consultant presents to clients that the impact of what their mind tells them is very quick and very automatic. From this perspective, mindfulness as an activity promotes a greater awareness of what the mind tells us as it occurs, and thus we can develop a greater capacity to control the choices we make in response to our mind's activity. The client is told that regular practice of mindfulness will first promote necessary self-awareness (and thus break the automatic process), followed by greater cognitive defusion (decentering from what our mind tells us), and finally the capacity to regulate attention as needed.

A useful metaphor that the second author has successfully used with clients is the parade metaphor. In this example, the consultant describes two people watching a parade. The first person finds a spot to sit and watches all of the acts as they come and go. Some acts are liked and some are disliked, but all come, stay a while, and leave, and a new act follows. Each act is experienced from beginning to end, and the person enjoys the full experience of the parade. In contrast, the other person sees an act that he or she finds interesting and spends the entire day following that act around, up and down the streets. The person gets frustrated bumping into people along the parade route and worrying about seeing the same act in the next location. At the end of the day, only one act was experienced, and, despite other acts being visible, the person was so worried about chasing the favorite act that the entertainment that was right in front of him or her was missed. Obviously, this person had a very different parade experience. Following an example such as this, the client is asked to consider living a more in-the-moment life. Both good and bad experiences will come and go, but the client can learn to experience life, as opposed to having a distorted and partial experience of life.

At this juncture, the consultant should briefly explain that a variety of mindfulness exercises will be utilized throughout the MAC protocol, and should also note that this and all subsequent sessions will begin and end with a brief mindfulness exercise.

DISCUSSION OF BETWEEN-SESSION EXERCISES: WHAT I HAVE LEARNED FORM, BRIEF CENTERING EXERCISE, AND WASHING A DISH MINDFULNESS EXERCISE

One of the key elements to the successful completion of the MAC protocol is adherence to the between-session exercises. At this point, the client is already familiar with the Brief Centering Exercise and has completed the What I Have Learned Form. During this session of Module 2, the consultant presents the next mindfulness exercise, known as Washing a Dish (see Figure 5.1). Instructions for this exercise should be handed out during the session and read together, with any questions answered prior to the end of the session. The client is asked to practice the mindfulness exercises at home six times before the next session, alternating between the Brief Centering Exercise and the Washing a Dish Mindfulness Exercise. A total of 6 days of practice is typically required (3 days for each exercise). Once again, this is presented as a necessary between-session exercise to promote the skill development and consequential benefits just discussed. We recommend that readers become familiar with the Washing a Dish Mindfulness Exercise before proceeding.

REVIEW SESSION

After introducing the Washing a Dish Exercise and reminding the client of the importance of between-session exercises, the consultant should review the session with the client. Important elements include recounting the concept of cognitive fusion (and defusion) and the relevance of self-awareness and mindfulness in the enhancement of athletic performance. Again, this presents an opportunity to emphasize that, for any skill to be developed, it is necessary to truly commit to practicing the skill. The consultant also should provide the client with the What I Learned Form, and discuss the importance of completing this Form as soon as possible

Washing a Dish Mindfulness Exercise

Choose a relatively quiet moment to select a dish and place it in an empty sink. Just look at the dish for a moment and become aware of the color, shape, and texture of the dish. You may become aware that other thoughts come into your mind while performing this exercise. This is inevitably going to happen because numerous thoughts come and go in our head all day, every day. Simply notice them, notice the tendency to fight them, and let them be. Gently bring yourself back to the task of focusing on the physical aspects of the dish.

Now, pick up the dish and allow comfortably warm water to pass over it. Notice the sensations of the water, its temperature, and the feel of the dish as the water passes over it. Once again, you are likely to notice a variety of thoughts unrelated to this task. If so, please notice without judging them as good or bad, right or wrong, but simply an activity in your mind that comes and goes like waves intermittently hitting a shore. The specific thoughts you are having do not matter, just your ability to notice and focus on the feelings and sensations that the water and the dish create. Allow yourself to feel the sensations in more and more detail. In this way, you continually strengthen your concentration.

Now, wash the dish with whatever mild detergent you normally use and become aware of the additional sensations of smell and touch that emerge from this activity. As you continue to mindfully wash this dish, notice any external sounds and any internal thoughts as though they are simply words or symbols on a ticker tape and gently bring your attention back to the task of washing the dish. Having a variety of thoughts is normal; be patient with yourself. The fact of the matter is the mind will always tend to wander. Remain in the moment with washing the dish and you will increasingly enhance your attention.

After about 5 minutes, wipe off the dish, stop the water, sit down and briefly describe the experience you just had in the space provided below. Include all thoughts, reactions, and actions that you took during this exercise.

Initials:
Date:
Time:
Place:

_____
_____
_____
_____
_____
_____
_____
_____

FIGURE 5.1   Washing a Dish Mindfulness Exercise

after the session. This is particularly important if the What I Learned Form was not completed the prior week. If the client had difficulty completing the form due to a lack of understanding of the purpose or instructions, the consultant can explain the form and directions for its use.

BRIEF CENTERING EXERCISE

Following the review, the client should spend about 5 minutes at the end of the session performing the Brief Centering Exercise again. During this exercise, it is important to help the client learn to tolerate feelings such as impatience, boredom, anxiety, and frustration as you slowly go through the exercise.

COMMON PROBLEMS SEEN IN MODULE 2: INTRODUCING MINDFULNESS AND COGNITIVE DEFUSION

The following are common problems with Module 2 that we have found when working with clients and during supervision of novice MAC consultants.

Lack of Consultant's Comprehensive Understanding of Cognitive Fusion, Cognitive Defusion, and Mindfulness

As was the case in Module 1, it is critical that the consultant fully understand the concepts presented and discussed in Module 2. For example, the consultant must understand the difference between the traditional cognitive behavioral model, which focuses on modification of the content of thoughts, and the acceptance model, which focuses on the modification of the relationship one has with thoughts. The role of the consultant is to: (1) enhance the development of self-awareness of thoughts as events (not literal truths); (2) promote the development of a decentered and nonjudging experience of thoughts; and (3) reduce the grip that those thoughts (beliefs) or emotions will ultimately have on behavior. The client is helped to understand that, with attention anchored, thoughts and feelings can be noticed as events that simply come and go and do not necessarily require action.

Mindfulness exercises function to promote a mindful state of being, which corresponds to the decentered experience noted above. It is only then that behavior can be directed not by internal rules or emotions, but rather by valued directions (to be discussed in subsequent chapters).

Hence, it is essential that both the consultant and the client understand the value of mindfulness practice and the central place that it occupies in the MAC program. Based on our experience, without this understanding, the use of mindfulness exercises will seem silly or irrelevant and may be used for incorrect purposes (such as relaxation). In fact, as noted earlier, the most common misconception about the use of mindfulness is the idea that it is intended to promote relaxation. Although a sense of peace and contentment often ensues with regular practice, the purpose of mindfulness practice is not relaxation, but rather a more complete and full experience of life. Relaxation assumes a need to alter or reduce in some way the experience of thoughts, emotions, and physical sensations. In contrast, mindfulness seeks to promote the idea that full experience and acceptance of internal experiences is the primary goal.

The consultant's ultimate goal in Module 2 is to provide the client with the clear perspective that all human activity occurs in the present moment, and only from enhanced self-awareness (mindfulness) can one choose how to respond to each and every challenge of life. It is often helpful to inform the client that the first step is to practice *being,* not *doing.* This is, in essence, the primary objective of mindfulness exercises. It is often most helpful for both the consultant and client to reflect on the distinction between mind*ful* activity and the mind*less* activity that so often consumes one's existence. Using examples such as driving a car, eating, walking, or even practicing/working in one's chosen field can be helpful in conveying this idea. A consultant struggling with this concept might consider remembering a session that was conducted in an automatic (mindless) manner, where the body was in one place while thoughts were somewhere else, as opposed to a session that was experienced in a focused, fully engrossed (mindful) manner. This concept is likely to be novel for most people (including consultants), and, as such, it is imperative that it be described and discussed in a slow, patient manner.

Clients Become Frustrated With or Do Not Engage in Between-Session Activities

It is essential that the issue of adherence be dealt with early and often in the MAC program. Issues of adherence are inevitable for some clients, either due to their own issues relating to behavioral commitment, a lack of understanding of the principles and purposes, or a perception of a lack of relevance of the MAC program. This is where the therapeutic relationship is most critical. Ultimately, the client needs to believe that the consultant is an expert and that the time spent engaging in these exercises will have a long-term payoff. This is particularly important in protocols that utilize metaphors and exercises that may not have an obvious point. For instance, in traditional cognitive behavioral therapy, the client usually completely understands the reasoning behind a thought record, but this same client may not intuitively understand the benefit of mentally washing a dish. Because some of the exercises seem a bit unconventional at first, the consultant should work hard to communicate the purpose of the exercises and the subsequent benefit that they will have on the client's overall well-being and performance. Yet, if there are problems in adherence, which will most often be noted from the absence of between-session exercise completion, we encourage the consultant to first focus on him- or herself before assuming a problem with the client. Have you clearly presented the material? Have you related to the client in a manner that conveyed a sense of understanding and compassion? Have you in any way conveyed mixed messages about the importance of exercise completion? Have you connected the purpose of each exercise to the ultimate goals of MAC, which in turn have been appropriately connected to the client's personal goals? Only after considering each of these questions should attention be turned to the client.

Reasons for client nonadherence can fill an entire volume. However, it is our experience that there are two common explanations for nonadherence: lack of commitment to the performance-enhancement enterprise and client perfectionism. These are the next two barriers to successful completion of Module 2.

Noncommitment to the Performance-Enhancement Enterprise

Despite their presence at MAC sessions, not all clients are truly interested in working to improve their performance. The client who is encouraged to participate by family, coworkers, coach, boss, or agent sometimes are going through the motions of cooperation without having a true desire to fully engage in the process. In addition, some clients want to enhance their performance but would like to do so with minimal effort or change in their approach. Issues such as these need to be carefully evaluated and directly approached by the consultant. It is our experience that, for whatever reasons an individual is present for the MAC program, there is always some "hook" to be found for them personally. The job of the consultant is to take the underinvolved client and find the reason for them to more fully engage. Without this time and effort, the MAC program is unlikely to manifest any significant benefits. It is not the consultant who has the magic bullet, but rather, the consultant must help clients find their own magic to enhance performance.

It may be necessary to ask clients to describe their approach to performance, and ask them to explain how it has worked for them so far. When the client says, "fine, I am truly happy with my performance," there is obviously nowhere to go, and engagement in MAC will not, and probably should not, occur. For these clients, there is no purpose for them to engage in the process, and a discussion of why they are present is warranted. In addition, it may be helpful to discuss with the client how he or she can effectively communicate the lack of intervention need with those who have insisted on attendance. However, for most clients, there will be some indication that their previous approach to improving performance has not worked very well. Clients should then be encouraged to discuss their efforts, which will often center on an attempt to better control their internal states (such as better self-talk, more relaxation, blocking out negative emotions, and similar control-based efforts). After clients describe these efforts and the limited success that they have had, the consultant should validate their experiences with comments to suggest that the problem is not that they have failed in their change-based efforts, but rather that the problem is the impossibility of the methods. That is, the effort to feel less and think better are doomed to fail because they are not consistent with the human experience. From this perspective, MAC is described again as an alternative that fits more rationally with the realities of life. As noted earlier, this approach is roughly equivalent to the "creative hopelessness" exercise that has been described in Acceptance and Commitment Therapy for clinical populations (Hayes et al., 1999).

The Perfectionistic Client

A number of clients truly desire enhanced performance but, due to their desire to be perfect in all ways and at all times, full engagement (and its associated risk of failure) can be problematic. For these clients, modifications of the MAC protocol are required, because high levels of perfectionism constitute performance dysfunction and therefore need to be addressed differently. For the mildly perfectionistic client, it is critically important that the concepts of cognitive fusion and cognitive defusion be emphasized. With these clients, the difference between actions required in the competitive moment (and in the service of valued goals) must be contrasted with the rule-governed behavior of perfectionism, in which choices and actions are made based on thoughts seen as realities ("I must be perfect," "I can't make a mistake"). Such cognitive content leads to inflexible and self-defeating behavior.

The following vignette illustrates both issues of noncommitment and perfectionism in a client who is a professional golfer:

CONSULTANT: I think we should discuss the lack of activity focusing on between-session exercises. What do you think is going on?

CLIENT: Well, I guess I have my way of doing things, and change is difficult for me.

CONSULTANT: Okay, tell me what you have done in the past to improve your performance and how well it has worked?

CLIENT: I read some things awhile back, and from these books I got into a habit of relaxing before competitions and repeating certain phrases to myself before each shot.

CONSULTANT: If that works for you, I wouldn't want to change things. So, tell me, how well has it worked?

CLIENT: (Laughs) I guess I haven't done it well enough, because I really haven't gotten any better. But I believe it can work, I just don't do it right, I guess.

CONSULTANT: How hard have you worked at it?

CLIENT: Very hard . . . but clearly I am not good at it, and I was hoping this program would help me get better at doing those things.

CONSULTANT: Okay, I understand. But what if I suggested to you that you probably do it pretty well? And, in fact, the problem is not you at all. The fact is, we know from research that the techniques you have been trying have only a very small success rate.

CLIENT: I know you said that in session one, but I don't know.

CONSULTANT: That's because you are holding onto the idea that you can fully control how you think and feel. But the human experience suggests that thoughts and feelings of all types simply come and go, and maybe your efforts need to be focused somewhere else. Maybe, just maybe, you can feel lousy and think crookedly sometimes, and still perform at your best.

CLIENT: I understand what you are saying, but it's hard for me to change because I am so concerned about making mistakes. I guess the things I have been trying may not have worked, but they're a comfortable ritual for me.

CONSULTANT: I agree, and I think that's a great insight. It seems that, like we talked about, when your mind tells you, "I can't fail" and "Maybe I'll screw up," you immediately act on it as though these thoughts are absolute realities.

CLIENT: There is no doubt that is exactly true.

CONSULTANT: Well, maybe we need to work on the idea that you can learn to see your thoughts as just passing events, like when you watch cars come and go on a highway. And then you can make choices based on what might be in your best interest, and not in the interest of satisfying your thoughts . . . like choosing to pursue some performance enhancement exercises that offer some hope, even though it causes some initial discomfort when your internal rules kick in. What do you think?

CLIENT: This is a very different way for me to approach things, but I guess since I'm here and I've made this commitment I should give it a try.

MODULE 2 CONSIDERATIONS FOR WORKING WITH CLIENTS EXPERIENCING PERFORMANCE DYSFUNCTION

As discussed at the end of chapter 4, the client experiencing performance dysfunction presents additional issues for the practitioner attempting to utilize the MAC protocol. The central issue in working with the client with performance dysfunction is the identification of the particular dysfunctional psychological process and not simply the *form* of the process. In the real world of practice, clients will frequently present with issues relating to worry, perfectionism, aggressive behavior, and numerous other psychological barriers to successful performance. Although the form of these difficulties must be recognized and understood, the practitioner should always remember that, ultimately, intervention must target the functions (or psychological processes) that underlie these difficulties. As an example, consider worry and perfectionism. Both manifest differently, although both involve strongly held internal rules (schemas) that guide behavior (rule-governed behavior). But the question remains, what is the function of these behavioral difficulties? Recent data from our lab offers some insight into the answer. In the study, it was found that experiential avoidance—that is, the desire to avoid internal experience perceived as in some way toxic (such as negative thoughts and emotions)—mediates the relationship between perfectionism and worry. It appears that the function of these psychological barriers is the reduction of personal discomfort through persistent efforts to avoid experiences that have been deemed to be unacceptable. Yet, the *long-term* performance-interfering consequences of worry and perfectionism become secondary to the *immediate* discomfort-reducing benefits. As such, the goal in working with perfectionistic clients or excessive worriers is the systematic promotion of values-directed behavior and the simultaneous reduction of emotion-reducing avoidance behavior, no matter what the form. Our experience indicates that most psychological barriers in clients experiencing performance dysfunction are, in fact, problems with various forms of experiential avoidance.

Because the goal of reduction of experiential avoidance is at the heart of MAC, the basic MAC protocol can be readily used with clients who have performance dysfunction who are, by definition, experiencing more significant psychological barriers. While performance enhancement is likely to follow as a positive consequence, it must be seen in the larger context of removing more pernicious pervasive forms of experiential avoidance, which will inevitably enhance the client's overall well-being.

CHAPTER 6

MAC Module 3:
Introducing Values and
Values-Driven Behavior

The primary purpose of Module 3 of the MAC program is the understanding and exploration of values as a central orienting concept. In the context of understanding the important role of values in enhanced performance and quality of life, the functional and dysfunctional role of emotions is also carefully considered.

In Module 3, the consultant first takes the client through an exploration of the important distinction between goals and values. It is necessary for the client to understand how achievement of *outcomes* in life is fundamentally different from the day-to-day *journey* of life. In the course of this exploration, the following questions must be asked and answered: (1) What do clients want their lives and their performance-related activities to be about? (2) What would they want teammates/coworkers to say about them in an obituary if they died tomorrow? (3) How do they want their lives and performance efforts and activities to be remembered? (4) What matters to them about their sport or occupation?

It is of critical importance that the connection between values and day-to-day actions and choices be the central feature of this module. Many clients remark that this module was the single most important step in the entire MAC program, and we believe that the primary reason for this is the presentation of values as an anchor for all future sessions. The client is led through the cornerstone idea that, by defining values and living a life that is directed by these values (including the performance-related components of life), they increase the likelihood that their performance goals will be met. The key to understanding this concept is in considering the alternative. The alternative to a values-directed life is an emotion-directed life in which one's actions are not in the service of what really matters to the individual, but rather are in the service of how the individual feels at any given moment. Although it is sometimes difficult to comprehend, the idea that living a valued life will ultimately enhance the likelihood that one's goals will be attained is central to the MAC program. Going forward, we suggest to clients that their personal values will be the anchor point for all behavioral decisions that need to be made in the course of enhancing performance and achieving goals. Based on this foundation, clients are challenged time and again to compare their behavioral choices to the values that they personally establish.

The question of personal values is particularly salient when confronted by the variety of emotions and internal rules that the client confronts on a daily basis. In this context, the role of emotion in human life, including the dysfunctional ways that it may guide one's moment-to-moment behavioral choices, is discussed in detail. The client learns to recognize and confront emotions *before* acting on them by posing questions such as, "Am I acting in the service of my values or am I choosing actions in the service of what feels good right now?" This allows behavioral choices to be made not based on internal rules or the emotions of the moment, but rather in a consistent values-directed manner.

Outline of Module 3

1. Brief Centering Exercise
2. Discussion of the What I Have Learned Form
3. Check for and Respond to Questions or Uncertainties Regarding the Previous Session
4. Discussion and Exploration of Values and Values-Driven Versus Emotion-Driven Behavior
5. Additional Home Mindfulness Exercise: Relevant Mindful Activity
6. Discussion of Between-Session Exercises: What I Have Learned Form, Performance Values Form, Given Up for Emotions Form, and Mindfulness Exercises
7. Introduction to the Mindfulness of the Breath Exercise

BRIEF CENTERING EXERCISE

As with each module of the MAC program, Module 3 begins with the Brief Centering Exercise. The intent is to continue to promote the regular use of this exercise, provide an opportunity to discuss the positive effects of its use, provide an opportunity to discuss any problems with its use, and create a centered, in-the-moment focus for the current session. After opening Module 3 with the centering exercise, the consultant should make the point that becoming mindful, or being in the moment, is more than simply an exercise. Rather, it is a state that requires ongoing and consistent effort. The consultant might point out that, at various points during any given day, the client will be able to notice that his or her head and body are not in the same place. This is ultimately the purpose of mindful activity. When this state is noticed, the client can gently focus on breathing and the physical realities and surroundings (using the senses to become aware of where one is and how one physically feels) to arrive at a place where one's body and mind are in the same place at the same time. The consultant can point out that this concept can be applied to a variety of performance situations in which the client is engaged, and the use of these weekly opportunities to enhance mindfulness can enhance concentration. This will become increasingly important as we move through the remainder of the MAC program.

DISCUSSION OF THE WHAT I HAVE LEARNED FORM

Similar to the purpose noted in previous sessions, the intent of the What I Have Learned Form is to monitor the understanding and assimilation of information from the previous module. The form should be collected and reviewed during the session. Again, failure to complete the form is processed, and the consultant directly responds to any questions or misunderstandings.

CHECK FOR AND RESPOND TO QUESTIONS OR UNCERTAINTIES REGARDING THE PREVIOUS SESSION

There are a number of common reactions to the Washing a Dish Exercise presented in Module 2, and the consultant may need to respond to client reactions and questions. Two examples follow:

1. Some clients report becoming frustrated during the Washing a Dish Exercise. Society often promotes doing things correctly, and this is especially common in high-performance domains. Thus, it can be perplexing to engage in an exercise that involves simply noticing thoughts, feelings, and physiological sensations with no goal other than becoming aware of these events. It is important to use this opportunity to promote the idea that the purpose of this, and all similar exercises in the MAC protocol, is to become

mindful (as opposed to mindless) by developing the capacity to pay attention, intentionally and nonjudgmentally. Although it may seem easy, it isn't, and normalizing the client's frustration and uncertainty is important to promote and reinforce further mindfulness practice.

2. Clients may report feeling bored during the exercise and may tell the consultant about the many thoughts that "popped" into their head. This will usually include all the important things that they needed to do but weren't able to do while engaged in this activity. Of course, this is exactly the point, and these types of comments are perfect opportunities to further elucidate why they are engaging in these tasks. These thoughts are *always* with us, and there is no need to make any effort to make them go away. Because this is a fundamental reality, the aim is to simply notice them as mental events that come and go all through the day (you can use the parade metaphor here), instead of seeing them as facts to which we must respond. Reinforce the awareness of these thoughts and the importance of gently bringing one's attention back to the physical object in question (in this exercise, the dish). This discussion can further clarify that *mindlessness* is those periods of time when our minds and our bodies are in different places (i.e., washing the dish but thinking about other activities), whereas *mindfulness* can be conceptualized as those periods of time when our minds and bodies are in the same place and are engaged in the same task.

Client reactions also allow for a discussion about tolerating an emotion (i.e., boredom) while still focusing one's attention on the task at hand. Having the client give an example of how this skill could be valuable in enhancing his or her performance is especially helpful at this point in the module. It should be stressed that the typical frustrations and difficulties with this simple exercise present the perfect opportunity to note the performance-enhancing effects of attention to task, even when competing thoughts and emotions are present.

DISCUSSION AND EXPLORATION OF VALUES AND VALUES-DRIVEN VERSUS EMOTION-DRIVEN BEHAVIOR

The work done to this point in many ways sets the stage for the next, and possibly most important, component of the MAC program: values identification. A sound understanding of the distinction between values-driven choices versus emotion-driven choices is critical to emphasize at this point of the MAC program. It is here that we begin to explore questions such as "What do you really want out of your competitive/performance experience?" "How do you want to be known and remembered by coworkers/teammates?" "What journey do you want to experience on the way to the destination you desire so much?"

The client sometimes wonders why the consultant is asking about such things in a program designed to enhance performance. Frequently, the client will answer the questions noted above by essentially restating goals such as "I want to be the best in the industry," "I want to be part of a championship team," or "I want to be as successful or as good as I always dreamed of being." It takes some effort to move these achievement goals into the context of values. Remember, the *journey* is the value. The *destination* is the goal. The first author uses the following metaphor to make this point:

Imagine having to drive cross-country to begin a new job. There is no need to rush, but, because you are excited, you want to get there as quickly as you can. So you drive nearly nonstop and you only stop for food, drink, minimal sleep, and fuel. You arrive in a remarkably quick time, and remember nearly nothing of your trip. You got to where you were going, but what of the experience? What did you see and what do you remember about the trip? What risks did you take by taking this approach to your trip? Now, compare that to the same trip, completed more slowly, with a plan to see and experience the country. You see things you never saw before and that you may never have the opportunity to see again. You took the time to experience the full measure of a cross-country experience. You still get where you are going, safely, on time, and ready to go to work, but you had an entirely different perspective and an entirely different life experience.

In discussing this metaphor with the client, there are two aspects on which to focus. The first aspect is the difference that each trip has on one's overall life experience. The second aspect highlights how the rapid cross-country trip was chosen as a direct result and in the service of the emotion of excitement, and was not in the service of life values and personal meaning. Either way, the individual gets where he or she is going, but each results in a vastly different experience.

At this point, it is crucial that this concept be brought back to the idea of performance enhancement. How does this fit? Are we suggesting that achievement goals must take a back seat to larger life values? The answer is no. It is our contention and our experience, both in practice and research, that performers who become focused on values that underlie their chosen competitive pursuits train harder and more consistently; make better choices, especially in the face of hardships and negative thoughts and emotions; and persevere in the day-to-day activities (i.e., training) that ultimately enhance the likelihood that they will achieve their goals. We believe that consistent, values-directed choices and behaviors (not emotion-directed behaviors) are the essence of the elusive *mental toughness* that athletes and elite performers want so badly to achieve.

> We define mental toughness as the ability to act in a purposeful manner, systematically and consistently, in the pursuit of the values that underlie performance activities, even (and especially) when faced with strong emotions that we as humans naturally want to control, eliminate, or reduce.

The following vignette, which immediately followed the presentation of the cross-country trip metaphor, highlights this concept to a would-be Olympic swimmer.

CONSULTANT: So tell me how you want to remember your swimming career.

CLIENT: I would like to win a gold medal of course, but I really do want to always look back and know I really put in the time and effort necessary . . . that I really gave it all I had. I would hate to look back and wonder "what if?"

CONSULTANT: How does this explain your recent practice issues?

CLIENT: (Laughing) I knew this is where we were going. Well, it doesn't. The days that I either blew off practice, or just went through the motions had nothing to do with what I just said.

CONSULTANT: Then how do you explain it?

CLIENT: I was pissed at my coach and just said, "Screw it!"

CONSULTANT: So those choices were based on how you were feeling about the coach at that time?

CLIENT: I have to admit it. It's like the story you told a few minutes ago. It had nothing to do with what I really, really want and everything to do with how I was feeling at that time.

In this brief vignette, the distinction between values-driven and emotion-driven choices is not only accentuated, but also elucidates the performance relevance of this concept. It is usually after the presentation of the trip metaphor that the consultant should either bring up known specific examples or actively search for new examples in the client's performance life that are related to this concept. This is not usually difficult to do and almost always brings home the point with great clarity.

At this point in the session, the consultant may ask the client to complete the Performance Obituary (see Figure 6.1) that is an extension and adaptation of the Tombstone Exercise used in clinical treatment by Hayes and colleagues (1999). In this exercise, the client is asked to write his or her own obituary as it relates to the competitive/work career. Essentially, the question is: how would they like others to remember them in this regard if they were no longer living? This experiential exercise begins the formal exploration and elucidation of performance values.

Upon completing the Performance Obituary, the consultant and client should examine the written material and cull the identified values that can be ascertained from it. These values should be remembered and referred to often throughout the remainder of the MAC program.

Following the completion of this exercise, we suggest that the consultant engage in a discussion regarding the function of emotion in human life. We suggest describing emotion as normal human activity that provides information (for example, the experience of fear tells us we need to act in some way to protect ourselves) and allows us to fully appreciate and experience our existence. In this context, love, joy, anger, sadness, and all emotional states allow us to fully participate in life. They allow us to *experience* life and not just have a life. Of course, emotions span a broad spectrum, as they can at times be painful and at times be joyous. Yet each contributes to our overall experience and should not be eliminated or controlled.

There are several issues relating to emotions in the context of human performance that need to be addressed at this point in the module. First, which emotions appear to be barriers or obstacles to the client? It is important that the consultant help elucidate which emotions are in response to which situations, and with what typical response. Much of this information should have already been determined through the pre-intervention assessment and case formulation discussed in chapter 3. It is important to be aware that, when answering this question, the client may present the emotion itself as the problem. Yet, in keeping with the basic conceptual foundation of the MAC, one of our goals is to help the client recognize the difference between seeing the emotions as the problem and understanding efforts to control or eliminate the emotion as the problem.

Performance Obituary

Initials_____ Date_____ Age_____ Occupation_____ Gender_____

What and how would you like your performance/work career and you as an athlete, attorney, salesperson, coworker, teammate, etc. to be remembered?

_____

_____

_____

_____

_____

_____

_____

_____

_____

_____

FIGURE 6.1   Performance Obituary

The following vignette presents a typical discussion of this topic with a high-performing mortgage broker:

CONSULTANT: So, what emotions do you believe interfere with your performance at work?

CLIENT: I guess anger and frustration, either with others or with myself.

CONSULTANT: Can you give me an example of a typical situation in which you get angry or frustrated?

CLIENT: Sure. This week is a perfect example. I have been working with a client for several weeks now, and every time I think I have it done—exactly as she wishes, I should point out—she changes her mind and I have to go back to square one.

CONSULTANT: And you get angry?

CLIENT: Hell yeah . . . I get off the phone and feel enraged.

CONSULTANT: And what do you do at that point?

CLIENT: I usually just sit there, think about what she keeps doing, and get even angrier.

CONSULTANT: How much time do you spend just sitting there?

CLIENT: I don't even know. More than I should. Then I go online and take a 30- to 60-minute break where I do anything but work, because I can't work when I'm that angry and thinking over and over about what a jerk she is. Of course, then I start to get pissed off at myself for being such a baby and realize that the reason I'm not more successful is my anger. Then I get depressed and will sometimes just take the rest of the day off . . . just like I did this week.

CONSULTANT: I'm a little confused here. Your client keeps changing her mind after you put in a great deal of work doing just what she asked you to do, right?

CLIENT: That's right.

CONSULTANT: Okay . . . then you feel angry? Why is that a problem?

CLIENT: Because then I can't work.

CONSULTANT: Well, hold on a second. How many people wouldn't feel angry or frustrated in a similar situation?

CLIENT: I don't know. Most of the people I work with just keep going when this stuff happens to them.

CONSULTANT: Does that mean they feel differently than you, or just that they respond to the feeling differently than you?

CLIENT: Good point. Never thought of that.

CONSULTANT: So the real question is, what is the problem? The emotion of anger or what you do when you feel anger?

CLIENT: I see what you mean. I can't deal with being angry.

CONSULTANT: So your choices then serve the purpose of making the anger go away and not continue to work.

CLIENT: I want to keep going but I just feel so bad.

CONSULTANT: Just like we have mentioned in a previous session. We want you to get to a point in which you want to keep working *and* feel badly, rather than want to keep working *but* feel badly. One sentence suggests that work and emotion can coexist, while the other tells you that work can't happen while in the presence of the emotion. How likely is it that you or anyone else can eliminate all emotions?

CLIENT: Good point. That isn't going to happen. But I just figured I had more of them than other people.

CONSULTANT: Maybe the issue isn't having or not having emotions, or even how strong those emotions are, but rather accepting the presence of emotions, even strong ones, as a normal part of being human and staying focused on what really matters to you. The difference is between actions that are emotion-directed versus actions that are values-directed. It seems like you just described emotion-directed actions as opposed to values-directed actions.

CLIENT: Absolutely. No question about it. That makes sense.

The second issue relating to emotion and human performance is the distinction between what has been referred to as "clean" versus "dirty" emotions by Hayes and colleagues (1999). A clean emotion is described as one that is directly and appropriately related to a given situation. On the other hand, a dirty emotion is one that comes from the learning history, language use, and idiosyncratic response that someone has to the initial emotion. For example, in the vignette just presented, the client had a clean emotion (anger) in response to a circumstance that most individuals would find somewhat frustrating (responding to the unreasonable behavior of others). However, in response to the emotion of anger, and following the avoidant behavior that he employed to reduce the emotional experience, it appears that overlearned self-schemas about self-worth and failure were triggered. These schemas in turn resulted in feelings of sadness. The secondary emotion of sadness was a response to the client's avoidant behavior triggered by the first (clean) emotion. In this case, the anger would be described as a clean emotion and the sadness would be described as a dirty emotion. The following discussion of clean versus dirty emotions is a continuation of the previous vignette:

CONSULTANT: There is one other thing I would like to talk about regarding the example you just gave me. It seems as though you respond to the actions you take to get away from the anger by becoming depressed. Is that right?

CLIENT: Yes. I really beat myself up for being so weak.

CONSULTANT: You mean weak for both having the emotion of anger and then escaping it by not working. Is that right?

CLIENT: Exactly.

CONSULTANT: Well, let's look at this a little bit more closely. We just discussed the reasonableness of feeling angry when responding to people that are not being reasonable. Other emotions are often reasonable in response to life events as well. Fear is common in response to danger, and sadness is common in response to loss, for example. We call those normal and expected emotions "clean" emotions. They are part of being human, and not only can't you avoid them, but, frankly, you wouldn't want to because they are appropriate and sometimes even positive. For example, joy in response to a positive event or love in response to someone we care deeply about.

CLIENT: That makes sense.

CONSULTANT: However, sometimes, somewhere in our own personal history, we are taught that some emotions are "bad" and not to be experienced. Feeling anger, for instance, is often seen as unacceptable. In addition, sometimes we learn from our life time of experiences that "failure" is unacceptable and bad, and when we think about our avoidance, we make it into the equivalent of failure and respond to the words in our head as though they are reflections of reality. We then experience the sadness over something that didn't really happen. For example, you didn't fail. You did avoid returning to work, and then didn't work hard, but your self-judgment and the words you used to think about yourself were just words, not realities. You experienced sadness in response to thoughts and images in your mind, not anything in reality. This is what we call a "dirty" emotion . . . an emotion in response to your internal reality, not the external one.

CLIENT: This is also connected to what we talked about last session, isn't it? You know, the idea that our thoughts are just thoughts and not reality.

CONSULTANT: Exactly. You felt angry, avoided work, thought about your-self as a failure, which to you was a reality, and then became sad.

CLIENT: I do that so much. My head is spinning thinking about how often I create a second emotion because of how I handled or didn't handle the first one.

As suggested in this vignette, the concept of dirty versus clean emotions is helpful in understanding the normality of emotion in everyday life and in recognizing the distinction between values-driven and emotion-driven behavioral choices. It should be clear that during Module 3, the con-cepts of mindful awareness, mindful attention, and cognitive fusion and cognitive defusion become integrated with the concept of values-directed versus emotion-directed behavior.

At this point in the session, the consultant should hand out the Given Up for Emotions Form and ask the client to complete it between the third and fourth sessions (see Figure 6.2). This form is intended to allow the client to explore the personal and performance-related con-sequences of expending unnecessary effort to control and/or eliminate emotions, as opposed to focusing on values-directed choices and actions.

After answering any questions about the Given Up for Emotions Form, the consultant should present the next between-session form to be completed. This form, called the Performance Values Form (see Figure 6.3), allows the client to explore and codify his or her personal performance-oriented values that will guide the remainder of the MAC program.

The purpose of both of these forms, to be completed between Modules 3 and 4, is to promote the identification of performance values and to explicate the distinction between values-driven and emotion-driven behavioral choices.

ADDITIONAL HOME MINDFULNESS EXERCISE: RELEVANT MINDFUL ACTIVITY

At this juncture of Module 3, the client has hopefully developed a better understanding of the importance of in-the-moment aware-ness and attention, and, as such, it is a perfect opportunity to pres-ent the next step of their mindfulness practice and development. The Relevant Mindful Activity Exercise is intended to connect the mind-fulness concept to a relevant performance situation in the client's life. For example, we have suggested that athletes engage in mind-ful stretching or mindful sport-specific drills (i.e., basketball lay-up

Given Up for Emotions Form

Initials_____ Date_____ Age_____ Occupation_____ Gender_____

The purpose of this form is to help you become more aware of what you have given up to reduce or eliminate your emotions. What opportunities in the service of your values are you giving up in the service of feeling less emotion? How is this affecting your ability to perform better and enjoy your competitive/work world more?

In the first (far left) column, list a situation related to practice, training, or actual competition/work that triggered a strong emotion. In the second column, write down the specific emotion that was experienced. In the third column, record what you did to reduce or satisfy your emotion. In the fourth column, write down what effect your efforts to control or reduce your emotion had on you. In last (far right) column, write down the long-term consequences of your efforts to rid yourself of these emotions (what you gave up to reduce or satisfy your emotion).

Complete form beneath example provided below

Situation or event	Emotion	What you did to control emotion	Short-term effect	Long-term effect on you
Criticized by coach	Angry and thought over and over about him being a jerk	Stayed quiet and took a "don't give a damn" attitude. Thought about friends	Felt less angry, but uninvolved the next day	Looked even worse in coach's eyes, didn't practice well, looked like I was pouting, didn't further my goals

FIGURE 6.2   Given Up for Emotions Form.

Performance Values Form

Initials_____ Date_____ Age_____ Occupation_____ Gender_____

The following is a list of performance values that may help direct your actions on a daily basis. After each value is recorded, please identify the barriers to, and the actions that must be taken in pursuit of, those values.

Teammate/coworker: What type of teammate/coworker do you want to be? What does it mean to be a good teammate/coworker? Why is being a solid team member/coworker important to you?

_____

_____

_____

Barriers and Necessary Actions:

_____

_____

_____

Sport/Work/Performance Activity: What do you value about your activity? The challenge? Prestige? Enjoyment? Getting to interact with teammates? Helping people?

_____

_____

_____

Barriers and Necessary Actions:

_____

_____

_____

Training: Is developing your skill important to you? Why is working at getting better meaningful to you? Are there any skills you'd like to learn or develop more fully?

_____

_____

_____

FIGURE 6.3   Performance Values Form

Barriers and Necessary Actions:

_____
_____
_____

Technical Skills: What issues or behaviors related to technical skill development do you care about (e.g., working on golf swing, sales presentation skills, etc.)? What would you like to do more of?

_____
_____
_____

Barriers and Necessary Actions:

_____
_____
_____

Tactical Skills: What issues or behaviors related to tactical skill development do you care about (e.g., planning a sales or presentation strategy, developing greater understanding of pitch or club selection, play, etc.)? What would you like to do more of?

_____
_____
_____

Barriers and Necessary Actions:

_____
_____
_____

Recreation/Fun: What type of activities do you enjoy? Why do you enjoy them?

_____
_____
_____

Barriers and Necessary Actions:

_____
_____
_____

FIGURE 6.3   Continued.

drills). The goal is to focus their attention on the specific sensations and experiences that are involved in these tasks, instead of engaging in the more typical automatic mindless task engagement in which the body is doing one thing while the mind is focused elsewhere. For business people, we have suggested that they engage in mindful interactions or conversations with colleagues in which they note the words, body language, and tone of their colleagues' conversation. This is in contrast to making quick assumptions about their colleagues' words, intent, and interest and subsequently focusing on their own upcoming response (or worse, focusing on something completely unrelated to the conversation at hand).

We typically allow the client to choose a relevant activity in which to mindfully engage, and we make certain that the goal is clearly understood by reiterating that we are working toward the development of a fully engaged, here-and-now focus of attention. We again stress the goal of enhancing the ability to observe and describe both internal and external experiences. If the client has difficulty choosing a performance-relevant situation, the consultant may suggest a nonperformance situation to try first. For example, mindfully eating and mindfully jogging are simple activities to practice real-life mindfulness skills. The most important aspect of this is to communicate to the client the goal of developing the capacity to be in-the-moment, nonjudgmentally and fully, to be able to recognize the tendency for the mind to drift away, and to mindfully re-engage so that body and mind are in the same place at the same time.

DISCUSSION OF BETWEEN-SESSION EXERCISES: WHAT I HAVE LEARNED FORM, PERFORMANCE VALUES FORM, GIVEN UP FOR EMOTIONS FORM, AND MINDFULNESS EXERCISES

It is at this point that the content of Module 3 is reviewed and the between-session activities to be completed by the client are discussed again to ensure understanding and enhance the likelihood of completion. It is particularly important for the client to understand the central role of values in the MAC program. In our experience, regular practice of MAC skills from this point forward is *critical* to ultimate performance enhancement. As such, Module 3 should not be completed until the client is truly able to comprehend the concepts, goals, and activities discussed thus far.

Mindfulness of the Breath Exercise

This brief exercise will help you expand your mindfulness skills and will allow for further development of mindful awareness and attention. This exercise should take no more than 20 minutes to complete. It is suggested that this exercise be completed at a slow pace.

Please find a comfortable sitting position. Notice the position of your body, particularly your legs, hands, and feet. Allow your eyes to close gently. [pause 10 seconds]

Take several deep breaths and notice the air going in and out of your body. Notice the sound and feel of your own breathing as you breathe in [pause] and out [pause]. Allow your focus of attention to be on your abdomen rising and falling with each breath. [pause 10 seconds]

As you continue to breathe in and out, imagine that there is a pencil in your hand and that you are drawing a line upward with each inhale, and then a line downward with each exhale. [pause 10 seconds] Imagine the picture that these lines would create. [pause 10 seconds]

As you slowly continue to breathe in and out, notice that you may become aware of a variety of thoughts and emotions that enter and leave your mind. Simply notice them as though they are part of a parade, gently allow them to pass, and once again focus on your breathing and all the sensations that come. [pause 10 seconds] Having a variety of thoughts and emotions is not incorrect or in any way a problem, but simply reflects the reality of the human mind. There is no need to change, fix, or attempt to control these experiences. Simply note the parade of thoughts in your mind and refocus on your own breathing. [pause 10 seconds]

Allow yourself to continue to breathe gently in and out, focusing your thoughts on the physical sensations of each breath that you take. Whenever you are ready, slowly open your eyes, become fully aware of your physical surroundings, and continue your day.

FIGURE 6.4   Mindfulness of the Breath Exercise

INTRODUCTION TO THE MINDFULNESS OF
THE BREATH EXERCISE

Module 3 ends with the presentation of the classic Mindfulness of the Breath Exercise (Segal et al., 2002), which is an extension of the Brief Centering Exercise. It is suggested that the client attempt to utilize this exercise in place of the Brief Centering Exercise when alone at home and when time permits, whereas the Brief Centering Exercise should be used when the client is in public surroundings and when time is limited. The Mindfulness of the Breath Exercise is described in Figure 6.4.

COMMON PROBLEMS SEEN IN MODULE 3:
VALUES AND EMOTIONS

We have noticed three common problems that occur with Module 3. Each will be outlined below.

Lack of Personal Understanding or Acceptance

By far the problem most likely to occur during this module comes from the consultant giving mixed messages with respect to values and emotions. It is in Module 3 that the concept of functioning at optimal levels while also experiencing the full range of human emotions is the central theme. If the consultant has difficulty either understanding or buying into this concept, the session is inevitably confusing and disjointed. Our experience in working with novice consultants, and even experienced consultants who have firmly adhered to the "change" agenda in the past (i.e., "you can perform better if you change your thoughts and feelings"), suggests that the consultant must personally assimilate this approach into his or her way of thinking and behaving in order for it to be applied successfully with clients.

While we have repeatedly stated this same idea in Modules 1 and 2, it takes on greater importance in Module 3, because the client is likely to have the first real opportunity to compare values-directed versus emotion-directed actions in the context of this particular session. Most clients have grown up with books, coaches, performance psychologists, and parents telling them over and over that they perform as they think or feel. The socially accepted view that you do as you think or feel can readily be seen in a news report during the NCAA men's basketball tournament, in which a surprise team made it to the Final Four. In the new reports leading up to the Final Four game, it was made known that a recognized sport psychologist (who is not a psychologist at all) met with the team during preseason and told them that if they *believed* all season that they could beat the preseason favorite to win the national championship, they actually could. The "think you can and you will" concept was given credit for the team's unexpected success and reinforces the notion—unsupported by any empirical evidence whatsoever—that performance is determined by the content of one's thoughts and feelings.

The MAC model asserts a very different message and is supported by a great deal of ever-accumulating empirical evidence. The message is simple: Successful use of the MAC program requires this message to be presented,

---

Performance, and in fact most human behavior, can occur regardless of the content of thoughts and feelings, as long as one stays focused on the task-relevant environment and continues to engage in values-driven actions.

---

demonstrated, and practiced; lack of understanding or anything less than full commitment on the part of the consultant is guaranteed to result in confusion and inevitable lack of success.

Absence of Client Examples

The second problem that is fairly common during Module 3 occurs when a less-than-fully-engaged client does not provide personal examples of problematic emotions and emotion-driven behavior, and, in response, the consultant either abandons the topic prematurely or simply continues to give his or her own personal experiences as examples. Via the elicitation and discussion of personal examples that highlight the concept, it is imperative to help the client develop a thorough understanding of and connection to the idea that optimal performance does *not* require thinking and feeling good. The absence of personal examples provided by the client may reflect a lack of understanding or may be the characteristic style of the more perfectionistic client who avoids providing "incorrect" information of any kind. Patience and careful consideration is required with both of these types of clients.

Difficulty Developing or Recognizing Personal Performance-Based Values

In a small number of cases, the client has significant difficulty identifying performance values. In some of these cases, the client has significant difficulty deviating from performance *goals* as their driving force. These clients cannot or will not allow themselves to see any purpose other than achievement of goals as a valid reason for involvement in their activity. In these situations, the consultant has to differentiate between unwillingness, which could be a function of a reactant (i.e., oppositional) personality style, and extreme success/achievement schemas. Both of these problem areas should have been noted in the comprehensive pre-intervention assessment and case formulation discussed earlier; if, for some reason, this assessment was not instituted, then the consultant is advised to select the appropriate psychometric instruments and evaluate the client for the possible presence of these issues before proceeding. If these issues are present, modification of the MAC protocol for performance dysfunction would be necessary and will be described later in this chapter.

In other cases, the difficulty in delineating values comes from a lack of understanding and some confusion about the concept. In these cases, some patient discussion and slow development of values clarification is suggested. This may require Module 3 to be split into two or more sessions. Consultants with less experience may find that Module 3 is best completed across a number of meetings rather than during a single session.

MODULE 3 CONSIDERATIONS FOR WORKING WITH CLIENTS EXPERIENCING PERFORMANCE DYSFUNCTION

When using the MAC approach with individuals who meet criteria for a classification of performance dysfunction (Pdy), a number of Module 3 modifications are necessary. First, however, it is helpful at this point to understand the core problem that defines the Pdy classification. Whether the proximal problem is excessive, albeit subclinical threshold levels of worry, anxiety, anger, some variant of perfectionism, or chronic inter-personal difficulties that interfere with optimal performance, there are some core behavioral processes that must be understood and ultimately addressed.

Attentional Narrowing and Lack of Emotional Clarity

Common to all anxiety- and anger-related issues is narrowed attentional awareness. In the case of anxiety and perfectionism, there is an excessive focus on the future in general and on future threat in particular. As a result, individuals experiencing these difficulties—whether at subclinical thresholds or meeting criteria for full clinical diagnosis—are not likely to respond easily to current contingencies that may facilitate optimal responses. In essence, they are so stuck in their head that they cannot see what is going on in front of them and around them. Rather, their attentional focus is excessively self- or future oriented.

Although such clients may appear to be a perfect match for the MAC protocol, they are likely to require more time for intervention success. This is because some of the basic processes required in the MAC program are particularly difficult for many individuals experiencing performance dysfunction. For example, in addition to attentional biases, these individuals also tend to have a difficult time detecting and differentiating emotions. Recent research supports this clinical observation. Several studies suggest that individuals with variants of generalized anxiety disorder report poor clarity and understanding of their emotions (Mennin, Heimberg, Turk, & Fresco, 2005; Novick-Kline, Turk, Mennin, Hoyt, & Gallagher, 2005). We have found that such MAC clients require a longer period of time to come to a full understanding and awareness of their emotions and typically respond more slowly to the benefits of mindfulness practice.

Emotional Experience May Be Amplified or Exaggerated

In addition to a narrowing of attention toward potentially threatening internal and external experiences, clients experiencing problematic levels of anxiety, anger, and perfectionism often respond with heightened reactivity to these experiences and subsequently respond with overlearned behaviors to avoid or escape these experiences. Recent empirical findings suggest that this pattern may paradoxically lead to an amplification of the unwanted internal states (Gross & Levenson, 1997; Turk, Heimberg, Lutarek, Mennin, & Fresco, 2005; Wegner, 1994). As a result, these individuals tend to have an even more difficult time accepting that the experience of emotion is not the primary problem, as they have spent a good deal of their life trying in vain to lessen or eliminate these experiences. It thus is likely to take somewhat longer for these clients to come to see the value of the acceptance-based approach of the MAC.

For such individuals, it may be necessary to utilize a technique known as creative hopelessness (Hayes et al., 1999), which we noted earlier in this chapter. In this technique, the consultant slowly takes the client through a discussion about all the ways that he or she has tried to reduce or eliminate the problematic emotion. None have been successful, and the consultant suggests that maybe it is not because the "right" or "best" approach has yet to be found, or that the client has not been good enough at efforts at control, but, rather, maybe the problem is the belief that control is even possible. It is then suggested that the client consider the possibility that the problem is not the emotions per se, but rather the efforts at controlling them. This can follow with a discussion of the costs of these efforts, in a manner similar to the Given Up for Emotions exercise described previously. It should be apparent that the MAC program is a comprehensive acceptance-based behavioral intervention that can certainly be utilized for clients meeting Pdy criteria. However, the time frame of intervention should be reconsidered for clients with performance dysfunction.

Rigid Patterns of Behavior

The third core problem that emerges with clients who have performance dysfunction is a rigid, overlearned behavioral repertoire that is primarily driven by avoidance and is highly resistant to change. These characteristics have not developed because they have been successful in achieving valued goals, but rather because they have been intermittently successful at providing short-term relief from the intensity of emotions noted above—thus their avoidance has been intermittently negatively reinforced. It should be pointed out that many avoidant behaviors are quite subtle. Many clients do not see their actions as avoidance at all, because the actions are so habitual that they seem to be automatic instead of chosen. In addition, it has been our experience that, even when such clients begin to engage in more valued behavior, they do so in a manner that still appears mindless. Rather than fully attending to and experiencing these activities, they experience anxiety, perfectionism, and/or anger, go through the motions of these activities and do not fully experience them, and subsequently do not connect with the external environment. In these cases, clients may report the events as though they were observers of their lives as opposed to active participants. The regular use of mindfulness, especially relevant mindful activity as discussed earlier in this chapter, can be of particular benefit for such clientele.

Our primary goal in discussing the more significant psychological barriers likely to impact the quest for optimal performance is to point out that, after careful assessment, clients experiencing performance dysfunction issues need a slower-paced intervention, and the consultant should take extra care to make sure that the intervention addresses the specific pathogenic processes each step of the way before moving onto the next sequential objective of the MAC program.

CHAPTER 7

MAC Module 4: Introducing Acceptance

The primary purpose of Module 4 of the MAC protocol is the development of an understanding of the costs associated with experiential avoidance. In addition, we highlight the contrasting benefits of experiential acceptance in pursuing performance desires within the context of a values-based life. The essential goal of this portion of the MAC program is to convey the idea that emotions per se are not the enemy of effective performance, but rather it is the things that people do to eliminate or otherwise control emotions that are counterproductive to high-level performance states.

During Module 4, the consultant and client explore the workability of the client's various efforts in the past to control negative thoughts, emotions, and bodily sensations. It is important to reinforce to the client that the lack of consistent success in eliminating or controlling emotions is not due to a lack of effort, the absence of the correct approach or strategy, or personal failings, but rather is due to the ultimate impossibility of this task. That is, the client must begin to recognize that many thoughts and emotions, both positive and negative, typify the human condition (including performance-related contexts) and thus cannot or should not be eliminated. All humans experience an array of cognitive content and feel a wide variety of emotions. Although all individuals experience occasional pain due to their thoughts and emotions, this pain typically pales in comparison to the suffering that individuals experience based on the assumption that such pain should not exist and the resultant efforts to minimize this pain in the present and future. A significant portion of Module 4 is therefore designed to build upon the discussions of Module 3 and help the client move toward an exploration of the costs associated with efforts to eliminate or control internal states. In this discussion, the consultant will detect and discuss the obvious and subtle ways in which the client seeks to avoid his or her internal experiences.

In contrast to behavior in the service of experiential avoidance (discussed in the previous chapter), the client is helped to explore the benefits of sustained behavioral commitment to valued directions, which often requires becoming more tolerant and *accepting* of internal experiences such as thoughts and emotions previously assumed to be bad, unacceptable, or painful. The client is presented with the potentially more powerful strategy of nonjudging acceptance of one's experience. As such, all of one's efforts can instead be applied to the task at hand, rather than struggling to control or eliminate thoughts and feelings. In the course of this discussion, the client begins to develop a new approach to the diverse thoughts, emotions, and bodily sensations that are experienced in the course of any type and any level of performance.

As previously noted, this approach is termed *experiential acceptance* (Hayes et al., 1999). It is important to clarify that this term does *not* outwardly suggest that all humans must simply accept unwanted life circumstances (although that at times this is, in fact, necessary). Rather, the term experiential avoidance is intended to convey a willingness to experience sometimes painful emotions in the service of pursuing performance-related values that are personally meaningful. The term acceptance also reflects the reality that negative thoughts, emotions, and bodily sensations are an inevitable part of life in general and of performance-related activities in particular.

Outline of Module 4

1. In-Session Mindfulness Practice
2. Discuss the What I Have Learned Form, Check for and Respond to Questions or Uncertainties Regarding the Previous Session, and Discuss Reactions to the Relevant Mindful Activity Exercise
3. Review the Performance Values Form and Given Up for Emotions Form and Pursue Discussion of Obvious and Subtle Avoidance Strategies
4. Experiential Acceptance as an Alternative to Avoidance and the Connection Between Willingness and Values-Driven Committed Behavior
5. Extending the Relevant Mindful Activity Exercise
6. Brief Centering Exercise

IN-SESSION MINDFULNESS PRACTICE

This module begins with the Brief Centering Exercise, after which clients are asked to engage in a brief "hearing exercise" in which they are asked to hear, without judging, the various sounds that may be occurring as they quietly sit. They are instructed to note the sounds, note any thoughts that these sounds may trigger, and then gently refocus on their breathing. After several minutes, clients are asked again to center themselves and finally open their eyes. As human performance of all types requires the ability to shift attention from external to internal and back again as circumstances dictate, this exercise is intended to advance the process of enhancing attention and concentration. By now it should be clear that each week mindfulness exercises are used in various ways to promote these skills for clients.

After this exercise, the consultant discusses the client's developing skill and experience with the Brief Centering Exercise and mindfulness in general. The frequency, specific times, uses, and outcomes of this exercise should be explored. By this time, the client should be using centering as a foundation to enhancing general mindfulness on a regular basis. In addition, as noted in earlier chapters, it is imperative that the consultant take special care to ensure that this exercise—and, in fact, all mindfulness exercises—are *not* used for the purpose of relaxation or any other means of control or avoidance of negative thoughts, emotions, or bodily sensations. Rather, mindfulness exercises should be used as a means of enhancing the capacity to observe and describe internal processes and external events. Of course, while engaging in the practice of mindfulness meditation, clients may experience an enhanced sense of well-being as a secondary benefit. However, its use is *not* intended to reduce negative affect and create a sense of relaxation. In the course of regular mindfulness practice, clients are expected to describe a new understanding of various emotions, express surprise at their reactions to various events, and make a variety of comments that signify a heightened sense of personal self-awareness. The absence of such reactions should be carefully assessed, because it may reflect a lack of true engagement in the mindfulness process.

Further, if mindfulness exercises are being performed with the purpose of enhancing the observation and description of personal experiences, clients should begin to experience a decentering from their thoughts and emotions (although they are unlikely to use this term) so that they distinguish these experiences as passing events that are separate from the self. In the context of mindfulness practice, it is also particularly important to discuss the idea of nonjudging acceptance of thoughts and emotions in this session, because it sets the stage for the development of an attitude of willingness to experience whatever occurs, regardless of its emotional valence. This is a precursor to enhanced performance.

DISCUSS THE WHAT I HAVE LEARNED FORM, CHECK FOR AND RESPOND TO QUESTIONS OR UNCERTAINTIES REGARDING THE PREVIOUS SESSION, AND DISCUSS REACTIONS TO THE RELEVANT MINDFUL ACTIVITY EXERCISE

Similar to its purpose noted in previous sessions, the intent of a review of the What I Have Learned Form is to continue to monitor the understanding and assimilation of information from the previous module. It is particularly important to ensure that the distinction between values-driven and emotion-driven behavior (highlighted in Module 3) is clearly understood by the client. As with all MAC sessions, failure to complete any of the between-session forms or activities is discussed, and any questions or misunderstandings require discussion.

In addition, it is important that the consultant discuss the client's personal reaction to the Relevant Mindful Activity Exercise. The consultant will review the activity chosen and discuss the experiences that the client had with this activity. Because this is the first time the client has attempted to move mindfulness into a real-world activity, it is imperative that this discussion emphasize the differences between mindful engagement in the chosen activity and mindless engagement in the activity. The distinction is often quite clear; clients who engaged in the activity in a mindful manner are able to share numerous comments and reactions, and those who mindlessly engaged in the activity provide comments suggesting that they completed the assignment in a rote manner and have little ability to talk about or discuss experiences. This distinction is particularly relevant in Module 4 (and all subsequent sessions), because clients are asked to incorporate Relevant Mindful Activity into increasingly complex performance-related tasks.

REVIEW PERFORMANCE VALUES FORM AND GIVEN UP FOR EMOTIONS FORM, AND PURSUE DISCUSSION OF OBVIOUS AND SUBTLE AVOIDANCE STRATEGIES

In this part of Module 4, the consultant takes the client through an elaborate discussion of avoidance; its subtleties as well as its overlearned and automatic nature; how it is negatively reinforced; and, most importantly, its costs. For most clients, conscious decisions to avoid unpleasant thoughts and emotions are obvious. However, individuals rarely truly understand the degree to which subtle avoidance strategies hinder their development (such as choosing to practice a more skilled and thus more pleasing activity at the expense of more challenging and often more important skill development). It is important for the consultant to investigate and discuss the obvious and subtle patterns of avoidance at play in the client's life. These patterns of behavior often interfere with the development of necessary skills (i.e., practice and preparation) and actual competitive performance (i.e., failure to make necessary sales calls, failure to take open shots). It is within the context of this conversation that the material collected in the Performance Values Form and the Given Up for Emotions Form are reviewed and discussed. The consultant helps the client see the difference between avoidance as an emotion-driven behavior and alternative values-driven behavior, which, by definition, often requires some experience of discomfort. As previously mentioned, we have found the use of a physical fitness metaphor to be useful at this juncture. In this metaphor, the consultant describes the necessary steps to achieve a high level of physical fitness: (1) deciding that the achievement of a specific fitness level matters for health, well-being, and attractiveness; (2) the decision to follow a specific plan of action (exercise, diet, etc.); (3) the daily choices required to follow that plan; (4) the willingness to experience discomfort and yet persevere when hungry or fatigued; and (5) the reality that many choices across many days, weeks, and months are necessary for the benefits to be reached. The client is asked to describe the various obvious and subtle avoidance strategies that may sabotage these efforts and the reasons for these strategies to be chosen. In this dialogue, it becomes obvious that short-term comfort rather than long-term benefit is the primary reason for most avoidance.

To help the client develop greater insight into the relationship between emotion, the avoidant behavior that sometimes follows the experience of emotion, and performance, the client is asked to complete the Emotion and Performance Interference Form (see Figure 7.1). The form asks the client to note the relationship between specific situations in which an emotion was present and how the emotion interfered with his or her performance. The client is asked to complete this form during the subsequent week with a promise of careful review and discussion to follow.

EXPERIENTIAL ACCEPTANCE AS AN ALTERNATIVE TO AVOIDANCE AND THE CONNECTION BETWEEN WILLINGNESS AND VALUES-DRIVEN COMMITTED BEHAVIOR

At this point, the session moves to an approximately 15-minute description and discussion of experiential acceptance and willingness as an alternative to avoidance. It is emphasized that acceptance and willingness are significantly related to the achievement of personal goals and values, whereas

Emotion and Performance Interference Form

Initials____ Date_____ Age_____ Occupation_____ Gender_____

Please record performance situations that occurred during the past week, the emotion(s) experienced, the degree to which these emotions interfered with performance, and how these emotions interfered with performance.

Situation	Emotion Rate Intensity 0 = none 10 = extreme	Performance Interference Rate Intensity 0 = none 10 = extreme	What Happened?

FIGURE 7.1   Emotion and Performance Interference Form

avoidance is inevitably connected to short-term control, reduction, or elimination of personal discomfort. Within the context of the physical fitness metaphor noted earlier, acceptance of discomfort and a willingness to experience this discomfort in the service of attaining personal values is highlighted. With a foundation based on Module 3's emphasis on values identification, this discussion is intended to lead to the beginning of a commitment to making choices and engaging in actions that are in the service of one's personal growth as a performer and as a person. It is important to again point out that this attitude might best be described as moving from a stance of "I want to perform optimally (and practice hard, work hard, etc.), *but* I am angry, anxious, or sad" to "I want to perform optimally (and practice hard, work hard, etc.), *and* I am angry, anxious, or sad." The Performance Values Form and the Given Up for Emotions Form may be reviewed at this time, specifically in this context.

Following this segment of the module, it is helpful to have the client think about a difficult or stressful performance situation and note the effect that thinking about this event has on the body. It is pointed out that these effects do not have to be eliminated or controlled. Instead, they should simply be noticed and allowed to coexist with the requirements of the moment. In essence, the consultant attempts to normalize internal events as normal aspects of both human performance and life itself.

It should be emphasized that the focus of this session is on helping the client develop and maintain *poise* (and thus a commitment to one's stated values) in the face of the inevitable emotions related to high-level performance activities.

We define poise as the ability to function (perform) as required and as desired *while* experiencing whatever thoughts or emotions are triggered by any given situation.

The presentation and discussion of poise from this perspective is central to the MAC protocol, and all activities up to this point have set the stage for this concept to be presented and understood. It is also the core concept that makes all between-session activities seem relevant. At this point, it is helpful to demonstrate how all of the exercises and between-session assignments come together. Attentional self-regulation, self-awareness, and decentering of one's thought processes through mindfulness practice; identification of performance-related valued directions; recognition of and willingness to experience emotions as normal passing events; and, finally, a commitment to act in a manner consistent with stated goals all coalesce at this point in the process.

The following vignette demonstrates how these concepts are tied together to make the case about poise:

CONSULTANT: So, let's summarize where we are at this point. In essence, we are suggesting that there are two interconnected foundations of elite performance, which are full attention to the moment and poise. How would you view the things you have been asked to do in relation to those basics?

CLIENT: Well, obviously, the mindfulness stuff is related to getting better at being attentive in the moment. And I guess having emotions and still being able to persevere toward what really matters to me is poise.

CONSULTANT: That's really good. All I would add is that emotions aren't the enemy of performance. They exist and will always exist for all of us. The key is noticing them and letting go, staying focused on the demands of the moment and maintaining the commitment to what matters in the long run.

CLIENT: It does make sense now why you asked me to fill out all those forms and do all those exercises. They were a pain and they took a lot of work, but they really did help.

CONSULTANT: You know, even in this work, the principles are still present. You are doing what matters, even if sometimes it doesn't feel good, in the service of something meaningful to you. You have really done a great job so far, so let's keep going.

EXTENDING THE RELEVANT MINDFUL ACTIVITY EXERCISE

Following a discussion similar to the one in the case vignette, the consultant again moves to the Relevant Mindful Activity Exercise. If the client previously had a difficult time choosing a simple performance-related activity from which to begin, it was recommended that a non–performance-related real-life activity be selected in its place (such as mindful eating). If that was necessary, at this juncture of the MAC protocol it is essential that the client move toward a performance-related mindful activity as noted and described in the previous chapter. If the client previously chose a relevant performance activity, the client should chose a higher level activity for mindful engagement. The following vignette of an elite-level soccer (football) player provides a good example of this process:

CONSULTANT: I'm glad you were able to use the mindful activity in your prepractice and prematch stretches.

CLIENT: Actually, it worked way better than I would have thought. I never realized how many other things I think about while stretching. And most, I have to tell you, were not related to football in any way at all. In the beginning, I spent a small percentage of time actually thinking about each muscle I was stretching. But each day I became more and more focused on the stretch. By the end of the week I was much more ready to work out. I'm not sure if the physical stretch was better, or I was simply more present, as you would say, and ready to go out and play. What I do is begin with the centering exercise and move right into the stretch.

CONSULTANT: Any day or time where it was challenging for you?

CLIENT: (Laughs) In the middle of the week I was pretty upset at the coach for some things he said the day before during a team meeting. When I got to practice the next day, I didn't really feel like being there. When I started to center and then stretch, I kept thinking about how angry I was. (Laughs) I was surprised how easily I was able to notice it, like we talked about, and just let it pass and move back to my mindful stretch. I really surprised myself. (Laughs) Not that I didn't think this stuff could really work. (Smiles)

CONSULTANT: Well that's great! It seems like you were really committed to your values and not just to feeling better. It seems to have worked just the way we would have hoped; maybe even better than we might have hoped for so early in our work together. Did you have to change anything in your routine in order to make it work so well?

CLIENT: Not too much. I only had to tell a couple of teammates to let me be during the stretch. It was surprising to me how much social chatter goes on during this time. So I just excluded myself by telling them I was working on a new pregame routine.

CONSULTANT: It sounds like it worked well. So, where do you think we can take this next? I mean, what football-related activity would make sense for you to try this with?

CLIENT: I've already thought about that, and I think I could try it on the drills we go through either at practice or before matches. Simple passing drills, which I know I do completely mindlessly, would be good place to begin.

CONSULTANT: That sounds good to me. It sounds like any of your drills would be a good place to go next. Think about what you want to focus on in the process, like the physical sensations of the ball hitting your feet or something similar. Remember, the goal is noticing and describing the sensations and not necessarily controlling them. Also remember that this includes any random thoughts or feelings you may experience.

CLIENT: I'm really curious about this because it seems to me that this is the essence of just playing: less thought and more action and reaction.

CONSULTANT: Exactly.

Clearly, in this vignette, the client has fully engaged in the mindful activity exercise and demonstrates a clear knowledge of the goals and processes involved. This example is provided not to suggest that all clients will be at this level of understanding or engagement, but rather to show the place the consultant would like the client to reach with this exercise.

The consultant should work with the client to determine appropriate and relevant performance-related activities to be mindfully practiced. It may help if the consultant keeps the following ideas in mind as these activities are defined:

1. Make sure that each activity is a small, incremental advancement from the previous activity. Remember, the goal is to systematically shape the regular performance-related use of mindful engagement in day-to-day performance activities.
2. Make sure the client has successfully completed the previous mindful activity and can express the frustrations, surprises, and outcomes of using the activity before moving on to more advanced activities. When in doubt, repeat the activity for another week. This is vastly better than moving too fast.
3. The activities should take clients closer and closer to mindful engagement in their sport or nonathletic performance activity. They should experience weekly success in this activity, and the practice of this activity should be framed as a clear manifestation of values-directed behavior.

BRIEF CENTERING EXERCISE

Since this is the midpoint of the MAC program, the consultant should take some time before ending this module to reinforce (to the maximum degree earned) the client's work and cooperation. The module ends with the Brief Centering Exercise, which should be quite easily completed by this time.

COMMON PROBLEMS SEEN IN MODULE 4

There are two common problems that we occasionally notice during Module 4. Each is described here.

General Lack of Engagement in the MAC Process Manifested by Absent or Inconsistent Follow-Through With Between-Session Exercises

Consistent noncompliance with between-session activities must always be carefully evaluated. In our experience with MAC, as with all psychological interventions, lack of between-session exercise compliance suggests one of two problems. The first subtype of noncompliance represents a lack of motivation for the performance-enhancement enterprise and is commonly referred to as *resistance* or *reactance*. This is typically seen in clients who are in some way forced or coerced into engaging in performance-enhancement efforts by staff, family members, or other influential parties. It is also found in clients who tend to be somewhat oppositional or resistant to the efforts of others to "force" things on them (as was discussed in chapter 3). While the issue of personal choice in making the decision to engage in performance enhancement efforts can and should be addressed early in the consulting relationship, the consultant often assumes (or even directly assured) that the client is motivated and ready to engage in the process, only to find out later that this is not the case. We strongly suggest that when performance-enhancement counseling is initiated based primarily on the desires of a third party, the consultant takes the time to carefully assess not only the client's motivation for the outcome of enhanced performance, but also his or her *commitment*. After all, motivation is simply the desire for something. Most performers do, in fact, desire enhanced performance, so the issue is not really one of motivation, but rather commitment. Is the performer willing to extend him- or herself for the desired outcome of enhanced performance? Is the effort that the client is being asked to undertake worth the anticipated outcome? Does the client believe that enhanced performance is really possible? How much is the client willing to sacrifice for enhanced performance, and why or why not? A discussion of these and related questions can occur at the beginning of the MAC program or when consistent lack of engagement is noted (this should be clear by Module 4).

The second subtype of client who demonstrates a lack of between-session follow-through is the client whose lack of follow-through directly reflects a *behavioral pattern* that needs to be corrected. These are clients for whom experiential avoidance *is* the primary problem. In these cases, the avoidance of between-session exercises reflects a core psychological process that must be addressed (this would reflect a performance dysfunction classification according to the MCS-SP). For these clients, avoidance is the typical way they deal with most aspects of life. Thus, their approach to the MAC program is not resistance (as it is for the first subtype), but rather reflects their general approach to life (and probably) their performance concerns in general. Responding to this client subtype will be explored in greater detail later in this chapter.

Mindfulness Becomes Associated With Relaxation and Affect Reduction or the Client Does Not "Buy" That It Is Okay To Experience Affect

We have stressed throughout the text that mindfulness must be presented in the context of describing and noticing the full range of thoughts, sensations, and emotions that are a natural part of the human experience. However, some clients have a difficult time accepting this concept. If this concern arises, we suggest that the consultant patiently move more slowly through the protocol and extend the seven-module format. Rather than viewing the MAC's seven modules as consisting of 7 sessions, the consultant should approach the MAC as consisting of seven distinct *segments* to be achieved as the client's acceptance and understanding of the concepts permit. This may result in 8, 12, or 16 sessions, and a new module should begin only after the previous module is successfully completed. Some clients will require more time to fully embrace acceptance as an alternative to control. This is especially true for those who enter the MAC program strongly believing that emotions and negative thoughts are bad and must be eliminated or controlled. These clients occasionally have a difficult time understanding and using mindfulness, understanding values-directed versus emotion-directed behavior, and developing a willingness to engage in activities that require a reconsideration of the role of emotion. Helping these clients see that the *struggle* against thinking negatively and against being angry, stressed, or anxious is actually the problem is critical for ultimate success with the MAC program.

We have previously discussed the issue of the consultant's comfort with and understanding of the basic acceptance model. This issue sometimes is related to a client's unwillingness to let go of the need to control and embrace an acceptance approach. If the client seems inconsistent in understanding or embracing the acceptance model inherent in the MAC program, the consultant should consider his or her personal understanding of the approach and how he or she communicates the messages contained in the MAC program. Watch for signs that a mixed or double message may inadvertently be communicated to clients. An example of this is provided in the following vignette:

CONSULTANT: Tell me about your experience with the performance-related mindfulness activity.

CLIENT: I really enjoyed it. When I got to work I was stressed out about the trial that was supposed to begin the next day, so I did my centering exercise, and then lined up my case notes mindfully.

CONSULTANT: How did that work for you?

CLIENT: Actually quite well. I became way more relaxed, which then allowed me to get my notes organized well.

CONSULTANT: I'm happy to hear that the mindfulness exercise worked for you.

Clearly, the client used the centering exercise to relax, and there is no evidence that the client engaged in her performance task mindfully at all. The BCE should have been used to notice and observe the anxiety, focus on the task at hand, and then allow the client to organize herself *while* feeling stressed. Rather, the use of mindfulness in this vignette reinforces the idea that performing well requires a reduction in stress, and further suggests that the BCE is an appropriate means to achieve that goal. This type of misunderstanding and misuse of mindfulness inevitably leads to inconsistency (at best) and frustration, disappointment, and ineffectiveness of the MAC program (at worst).

MODULE 4 CONSIDERATIONS FOR WORKING WITH CLIENTS EXPERIENCING PERFORMANCE DYSFUNCTION

Module 4 may require several modifications for individuals meeting criteria for a classification of performance dysfunction (Pdy).

The first modification, noted above, is the possible need to extend the number of sessions from seven to a more flexible number determined by the needs of the client and the training and experience of the consultant. This is necessary for clients whose level of experiential avoidance is particularly problematic (thus making the regular practice and appropriate use of mindfulness difficult) and when there is inconsistent engagement in the acceptance agenda. Many clients experiencing subclinical levels of anxiety, anger, stress, worry, or perfectionism will begin to see the futility of, and begin to question the cost of, previous efforts at control. However, they may be hesitant to accept or willingly experience their internal states for fear that it may suggest resignation or defeat. For many such clients, acceptance also seems contrary to what they have been taught and have strongly believed for so long. The consultant is advised to constantly check for and correct any misconceptions that the client may have about the nature of experiential acceptance. We again present the idea that mindfulness and acceptance means letting go of the need to change things that are noticed (such as thoughts or feelings). The client with performance dysfunction must be encouraged to recognize that noticing an internal experience, without making an effort to change the experience, is *not* "giving in" or "giving up." In actuality, it is a process of letting go and moving on. We are not asking the client to cling to experiences (even negative ones), but are promoting a willingness to allow these experiences to occur naturally in the course of living a valued life.

Clients with performance dysfunction should be patiently helped to see that acceptance entails a willingness to see things as they are in the moment. It does not mean that they have to like what they see or become passive about life; it means seeing what is, as it is right now. Acceptance begins with the stance of accepting what you already have, thinking a thought as it comes to mind, feeling a feeling as it arises, and acknowledging this reality. As an example, consider a situation in which an individual was berated by a boss or coach. Even if it was unfair that he or she was berated, the individual must accept the reality (including his or her personal reaction) in order to effectively move through and beyond the moment. This stance keeps the individual from being stuck in, and in turn responding to, the host of thoughts and feelings that may be understandable but that do not reflect the needs and demands of the situation at hand.

Another example we share with performers is the idea that taking risks means feeling vulnerable. Having such feelings does not mean that risk-taking behaviors must be avoided and that one should resign to present circumstances. Rather, when the performer allows the vast array of thoughts, emotions, and bodily sensations to emerge as she or he engages in actions that are relevant and meaningful, she or he is able to function beyond the artificial limits imposed to avoid the experience of discomfort.

For many clients, this new way of responding to and dealing with the world is confusing and scary. While previous efforts to control and limit thoughts, feelings, and sensations have probably not consistently worked, they are, on occasion, effective and thus create an intermittent schedule of reinforcement that can be difficult to change. As such, we caution the consultant to take the time that is needed with these clients and patiently persist in the efforts to explain the model and engage the client in an acceptance agenda.

Showing compassion for clients struggling with letting go of the control agenda is particularly important. When clients experiencing Pdy-related concerns begin to practice mindfulness, they often report many critical thoughts and judgments about their internal experiences (e.g., "I shouldn't be worrying so much," "I don't know if I am doing this well enough") and their satisfactory completion of between-session exercises ("I'm not doing this right," "I don't get it"). The consultant has an opportunity to help the client be compassionate toward him- or herself by sharing his or her own personal struggle with mindfulness and acceptance.

Remember, what we are doing is changing the way that clients relate to their internal experiences. We are *not* attempting to change the experience itself. This process is difficult for many clients and requires patience and understanding on the part of the consultant.

For some clients, acknowledging the degree to which they have avoided in the service of reduced emotion and greater comfort is difficult. These clients may become upset by the assertion that it is okay to have negative feelings. Comments such as "Sure, it's easy for you to say, you don't have to feel this way" are common. It is essential that the consultant patiently engage this behavior with some appropriate self-disclosure (e.g., essentially communicating the fact that we all have to deal with separating how we feel and what we do) in order to reduce the implication that the client's problem in some way reflects deficits or weaknesses. The process of breaking a pattern of avoidance and enhancing a pattern of willingness requires slow and careful exposure-based assignments requiring gradual and steady steps toward facing and experiencing emotions that were previously considered unacceptable and/or frightening.

As suggested earlier, we cannot stress enough the importance of carefully assessing for the presence of Pdy-related issues prior to beginning the MAC protocol. Taking the time to appropriately and effectively assess for these issues can decrease program length, reduce client frustration, and dramatically increase the likelihood of intervention effectiveness for this subgroup of performers.

CHAPTER 8

MAC Module 5: Enhancing Commitment

The first four modules of the MAC program focus mainly on the development of mindfulness as a means of self-regulating attention and decentering from one's own internal experience; values identification as a means of determining the direction clients would like their actions to take them; and the development of poise (experiential acceptance as opposed to experiential avoidance) as a necessary element in the attainment of those valued directions. Beginning with Module 5 of the MAC protocol, we seek to enhance the client's *commitment* to attaining performance-related values through the activation of specific values-directed behaviors. In this portion of MAC, the intent is to again help clients distinguish between goals and values and explicate specific behaviors that will optimize what really matters to them in their individual performance domain.

In the first segment of Module 5, the client and consultant revisit how greater attention to one's present moment experience (promoted by the use of mindfulness) can foster more consistent and effective performance. We also review the role that emotion plays as a barrier against necessary performance behaviors and, conversely, the concept of poise as a necessary ingredient in optimal performance. We then briefly revisit the difference between values and goals and provide more detail than was given earlier in the MAC sequence. Finally, we identify specific behaviors (e.g., more intense and/or quality practice time, more time spent on skill development and tactical/strategic knowledge) that, if engaged in regularly and consistently, are likely to result in enhanced performance. It is essential that the consultant view his or her task in Module 5 as the identification of the *specific behaviors* that are most likely to directly and indirectly result in the meaningful enhancement of the client's performance life. This can include: (1) practice and/or training-related behaviors (specific behaviors related to greater intensity, greater involvement, greater commitment of time); (2) team-oriented behaviors (specific behaviors related to interpersonal effectiveness and communication); and (3) direct competitive behaviors (specific behaviors related to aggressive competitive actions, appropriate risk-taking in the service of improved effectiveness). The key is the activation of the specific behaviors related and connected to the valued directions previously identified.

It is important that the consultant point out and discuss during this and all subsequent MAC sessions the array of thoughts and emotions that can be (and often have been in the past) barriers to the ongoing commitment to necessary performance behaviors. This ongoing discussion allows the client to regularly connect with the material discussed in previous sessions and promotes a sense that the material in each of the MAC modules is intertwined. During Module 5, it is common for clients to suggest that the sessions seem to be merging together and that clear differentiation between topic areas becomes more and more arbitrary.

Outline of Module 5

1. In-Session Mindfulness Practice
2. Review of Previous Session
3. Enhancing Commitment: Connecting Values, Goals, and Behaviors
4. Review and Assign Performance-Relevant Mindfulness Homework
5. Session Review and Brief Centering Exercise

IN-SESSION MINDFULNESS PRACTICE

As with all MAC modules (and individual sessions), Module 5 begins with the Brief Centering Exercise. This provides another opportunity for further skill training as well as an opportunity to continue the discussion of the uses and benefits of regular mindfulness practice. After several minutes of the BCE, the client is asked to open his or her eyes, choose an object in the room or out a nearby window, and engage in a "seeing exercise" in which the client is asked to focus on specific aspects of objects (color, texture, shapes, etc.) without labeling the objects. For example, instead of saying, "an oil painting on the wall," the client will instead report that he or she sees a square, rough-textured object of yellow, brown, and orange colors. Following this brief seeing exercise, the client is asked to close his or her eyes and recenter before opening the eyes again. This exercise is intended to promote attentional flexibility and present-moment awareness.

By now, the regular use of mindfulness should be in place, the benefits verbalized, and the barriers substantially reduced. If this is not the case, it is imperative that as much time as necessary be set aside to discuss the obstacles and to develop a strategy that will help the client move ahead with this core skill.

REVIEW OF PREVIOUS SESSION

Early in Module 5 (as in all MAC modules), the consultant reviews the material covered in the previous session. This is of particular importance at this point in the program, because successfully enhancing commitment is based on the adequate assimilation of concepts relating to the willingness to experience emotion in the service of personal values (experiential acceptance). In fact, a great deal of new information has been presented to the client since the beginning of the MAC program. By this point, the client should understand the role of attention in optimal performance and the role of mindfulness in enhancing attentional skills. The client also should understand the value of mindfulness as a means of decentering, or becoming an objective observer of his or her own thoughts and emotions. The client should by now have delineated his or her personal performance values and should understand how acting in the service of emotion can at times be a barrier to the attainment of these values. In addition, the distinction between emotion-driven behaviors and values-driven behavior should now be fully understood by the client. Taken together, this is a great deal of new information and new skill sets. The consultant should, therefore, take some care in reviewing previously presented material and should respond to any questions or uncertainties that may still exist. During the review of MAC concepts, the consultant should not simply focus on the client's understanding of discrete concepts, but should look for the *integration* of previous concepts. Of course, the consultant will take time to provide additional guidance and discussion when necessary. We typically find that clients have a fairly solid understanding of the components presented in Modules 1 through 4, and that early in Module 5, a quick and simple review to tie the components together has a beneficial result.

An important component of this review is a discussion of the Emotion and Performance Interference Form that was handed out during Module 4. In the course of this discussion, the consultant will carefully go through the form and discuss with the client each situation recorded. In particular, it is important that the client be able to connect the ways in which a specific emotion led to a negative performance impact. Clients will typically struggle to understand *how* the emotion led to negative performance outcomes. They may recognize, for example, that anger or anxiety led to reduced performance on Tuesday afternoon, but may find it hard to explain exactly why. This is typically because most of us have learned to ascribe the emotions themselves as the *reason* for much of our problematic behavior. For example, "I was angry, so I did X," or "I was anxious, so I didn't do Y." Both examples infer that the affect is the reason for behavioral outcomes. Most people need help to recognize that the behaviors they engage in and the choices they make when experiencing emotion are the *real* causes of performance decrements. For example, the client may report, "I became frustrated, so I couldn't concentrate and I didn't make the sales call I needed to make," or "I was so anxious about screwing up that I made excuses so that I didn't have to get out there and give it a shot." In each statement, the unstated blame for the problematic performance behavior is on the emotional state. We want to help the client see the choice points where emotion-directed actions as opposed to values-directed actions are occurring. These are the *real* reasons for performance difficulties. In these examples, it also can be helpful for the consultant to point out ways that the use of MAC's core skills such as mindfulness and experiential acceptance can be of value in this regard. The consultant and client will be able to see the extent to which the client blames emotions for direct performance decrements by scanning the "how it interfered" column of the Emotion and Performance Interference Form. During Module 5, the client should soon reach the point at which the "how it interfered" column will be blank as he or she develops greater experiential acceptance and values-driven behavior and rejects the previously held belief that emotions are the cause of performance difficulties. Eventually, this form will become unnecessary, because over time the client will be increasingly able to disconnect performance behaviors from emotions—a fundamental goal of the MAC program.

ENHANCING COMMITMENT: CONNECTING VALUES, GOALS, AND BEHAVIORS

By now, the client has developed a solid idea of what he or she wants the performance life to be about, what he or she needs to do to perform more optimally, and what barriers are likely to arise. Now, the intent is to activate clients in the direction of a deep and ongoing commitment to consistently engaging in the actions and activities that are likely to give them what they want from their performance endeavors. Essentially, we now ask our clients to commit to doing what is necessary to enhance their performance.

Helping clients differentiate between motivation and commitment is a valuable tool here. We suggest that *motivation* is simply the desire for something. All people are motivated. And most individuals are motivated to perform better at whatever they do in love, work, and play. However, far fewer people are actually *committed* to doing the things necessary to perform better.

Commitment is demonstrated when one regularly and consistently demonstrates the specific behaviors and activities that are likely to directly result in optimal performance.

Here, we ask the client an important question. We ask if the client is ready to do what is necessary for optimal performance and the pursuit of his or her personal performance values. Of course, we reiterate that we are asking them to commit to this work even in the face of unpleasant internal experiences. The client is encouraged to accept these experiences just as they are (good or bad, pleasant or painful) instead of how they wish them to be or how they interpret them to be. The commitment to enhanced performance requires a yes or no answer to the question and requires the realization that life will ask this question over and over again, each day, and through each frustration and difficulty. Revisiting a phrase earlier in the text, the question can be asked, "Are you willing to commit to the values you have previously defined *and* accept whatever discomfort your mind and body experience along the way?" We emphasize to the client that the choice is clear. The client can either sacrifice the performance life he or she wants in an endless and ultimately futile attempt to struggle with and control thoughts, feelings, urges, memories, and physical sensations, or the client can choose to experience the varying array of internal experiences that inevitably occur while consistently acting in the service of performance values.

With the stage set, the consultant now introduces the Committing to Performance Values Exercise (see Figure 8.1). In this exercise, the client:

1. Connects values to both short- and long-term goals.
2. Connects goals and values to specific behaviors that are in need of addition or a change to promote those goals and values.
3. Regularly monitors naturally occurring situations that require some action in the service of the goals and values.

When first introduced during Module 5, the Committing to Performance Values Exercise should be reviewed by the client and consultant together, perhaps using a recent situation as an example. The client is then asked to complete the form between sessions to both monitor events and the presence or absence of behaviors identified as necessary for the attainment of stated values.

Committing to Performance Values Exercise

Initials_____ Date_____ Age_____ Occupation_____ Gender_____

Performance Value (PV):

_____

Short-Term Goal Associated With PV:

_____

Long-Term Goal Associated With PV:

_____

Behavior To Be Added or Changed To Achieve PV:

_____

Situation:

_____

_____

Action Taken:

_____

_____

Situation:

_____

_____

Action Taken:

_____

_____

FIGURE 8.1   Committing to Performance Values Exercise

The following vignette provides an example of how this exercise can be introduced and used to define and promote the activation of behaviors in the service of performance values.

CONSULTANT: So let's get down to it. When we discussed performance values a couple of weeks ago, you mentioned two. The first was to maximize your collegiate athletic experience so you can remember it well and be remembered well by teammates and coaches. The second was to put forth maximum effort so you get the most out of whatever ability level you have. Does that sound about right?

CLIENT: Yep. I've thought of those things a lot since that session, and I really want to make sure I get the most out of the experience. I want to be a good teammate and help my team win, and I want to be as good as I can be personally.

CONSULTANT: So let's break this down a little bit. Let's start with your performance value of enjoying the experience and being a good teammate, and then we'll move to the second performance value of maximizing your effort and getting the most out of yourself.

CLIENT: Sounds good.

CONSULTANT: Good. Let's take a look at this form. We call it the Committing to Performance Values Form. Why don't you write in your first performance value at the top. Great. Now, let's talk about the long-term goals that are associated with this value. What do you think those might be?

CLIENT: Well, as a good teammate, I guess my relationships with the other guys on the team would be solid, and I think that if we all acted that way we would be way better as a team.

CONSULTANT: Okay, so you are saying that both personal relationships and team performance may be enhanced if you continuously act in a committed manner toward that value.

CLIENT: Yeah, I think that's true.

CONSULTANT: So let's write that down. Now, what might the short-term goals be?

CLIENT: I'm not sure.

CONSULTANT: Okay. Think about it for a minute.

CLIENT: (Long pause) I think a short-term goal might be better communication between me and my teammates and more fun on and off the court.

CONSULTANT: Great. Now write that down. Okay, now we get to maybe the most important part of this exercise. Think about what *specific* behaviors or actions, in the service of this value, you would have to exhibit more or less frequently than you now do in order for these short- and long-term goals to occur?

CLIENT: Actually, that's pretty easy. I'd have to complain less about some teammates (laughs), reach out and be more involved on and off the court with teammates, and really make a better effort at communicating and being upbeat at every practice. I'd make each practice important and each teammate feel like I want to feel. I think I have a real bad habit of getting real quiet and noninvolved at practice. It's gotten me into trouble with coaches and makes them think I have a bad attitude and am lazy, and some teammates who think I dog it when I don't feel like practicing.

CONSULTANT: Are they right?

CLIENT: Maybe they are. No. I know they are.

CONSULTANT: Okay then. Let's write it down. Now, the next part is all up to you, just the way we have been talking about it. You have just identified what you need to do in the service of your goals. In the next sections of the exercise, which you'll complete during the week, you should take one or two situations that occur during the week that involve this area and record it. What the situation is and what you did. This will record your committed actions, and it will be the beginning of living a performance life directed to getting what you really want. Then we'll review this form next week, and each week after that.

CLIENT: Let's see how I do.

CONSULTANT: I am sure you'll do just fine. Remember, if being the best you can be really matters, then putting effort into this is just another part of that journey. Let's spend a couple of minutes reviewing the barriers that you might face and how you can use the skills we have gone over the past few weeks to help you be most effective.

CLIENT: Okay.

CONSULTANT: So, what might get in the way of you doing what you are setting out to do here?

CLIENT: Well, in the past it was always getting angry or frustrated. I'd get pissed at someone or something, and sort of say, "what the hell" and then just go through the motions. My attitude was, "it's only practice." But, then came game time and if I got pissed off, then I would just keep thinking about it over and over, and get out of my game.

CONSULTANT: Let me first point out to you, again, that you have made it seem here as though the anger or frustration *does* things to you, when, as we have talked about, in reality, you make a choice to *act* on the anger and not on what really matters. Anger is just an emotion—not good or bad; it just is—and it always comes and goes. So, how are you going to handle it in the future? Because you know for sure that at times you'll definitely get angry or frustrated.

CLIENT: (Laughs) Yeah, you keep telling me that. I guess I understand, but sometimes it's so automatic. I know I have to just have it, as you would say, and just let it pass, like I do with a lot of the thoughts I have during the mindfulness work. Just let it pass and refocus on what I need to do.

CONSULTANT: Pretty confident that you'll do it?

CLIENT: I probably won't always, but way more than I have in the past.

CONSULTANT: I can't ask for more than that . . . and how will doing this contribute to your values?

CLIENT: Oh man, more than anything else I can think of.

CONSULTANT: Well, I have faith that you'll work hard to do the things that will contribute so strongly to your values.

This vignette begins with values delineation and progresses through the establishment of both short- and long-term goals associated with those values, specific behaviors to be the focus of attention, and finally a brief discussion of likely barriers. The client is asked to complete this form for as many situations as necessary related to the first performance value identified. In some cases, during this same session, a second performance value will be identified, and the entire form will be completed in the same manner. In the beginning of the vignette, a second performance value was noted and would therefore have been discussed next. It may take more than one session to fully complete the form, with additional performance values added later. As illustrated by the vignette, the prime goal is to set the stage for the activation of performance-specific behaviors related to the client's values and goals.

Finally, in this section of Module 5, some clients will need help in developing a strategy for how, where, and when to engage in these new behaviors. The consultant should be aware that adding new behaviors or reducing the frequency of old ones is not always an easy task. Thus, some discussion regarding how, when, and where may be necessary to enhance the likelihood of success.

REVIEW AND ASSIGN PERFORMANCE-RELEVANT MINDFULNESS HOMEWORK

The first issue the consultant should address in this section of Module 5 is the question of whether the client has been able to successfully complete the previous mindful activity and can openly express the frustrations, surprises, and outcomes of using the activity. This is important to address before moving on to more advanced relevant mindful activities. By now, it is assumed that the client has adopted a fairly regular practice of mindfulness, which should include centering exercises and a variety of relevant mindful activities. Of course, this assumption should be checked directly. If regular and consistent mindfulness practice is not occurring, the reestablishment of this practice must take precedence. It must always be emphasized to the client that regular and ongoing mindfulness practice is a core component of performance enhancement efforts, and its regular practice is as important as any other aspect of the client's training and preparation.

At this time, the practice of relevant mindful activities should be taking the client closer and closer to mindful engagement in his or her athletic or nonathletic performance activities. The client should experience weekly success in this activity, and the practice of this activity should be framed as a clear manifestation of values-directed behavior. For example, mindful stretching can now move to mindful engagement in drills and then to mindful engagement in other relevant aspects of practice. The regular use of centering and mindful breathing may now be used just before competition and during naturally occurring breaks during competition.

In Module 5, the consultant continues to help the client move ever closer to mindful engagement in competition by focusing more heavily on mindfulness practice. Obviously, how this is applied will vary based on the performance activity, the particular performer, and his or her growing comfort with and confidence in mindfulness exercises. The consultant and client will clearly have to work together in a collaborative and creative manner to most appropriately apply mindfulness practice to the specific performance activities in question. Some examples from our professional work have included:

- Mindful sales presentation practices prior to the "real thing."
- Mindful lay-up drills before practice and a game.
- Mindful hockey passing and shooting drills just before a game.
- Mindful warm-ups for a baseball pitcher both between starts and just prior to a start.
- Mindful engagement in conversation with an executive during a board meeting.

- Mindful foul-shooting during practice.
- Mindfulness of the swimming stroke during long-distance swimming practices.
- Mindful practice of a closing argument in front of associates just prior to the completion of a trial.

What is common to all of these performance-relevant mindfulness exercises is the use of centering and mindful breathing to allow the performer to be fully present in the moment. We want the client to note thoughts and feelings as they arise but allow them to pass and remain focused on, and committed to, the full experience of the physical and/or mental task at hand. Going back to the model of functional and dysfunctional performance discussed in chapter 1, this mindfulness activity allows the performer to remain task-focused even in the face of random thoughts and emotions that would otherwise occupy and distract. We have been asked if such total engagement in the moment—including the noting of thoughts and emotions—isn't, in fact, a form of self-focused attention. Our answer is that the awareness of naturally occurring thoughts and feelings is not equivalent to self-focused attention. True self-focused attention is the effort to control or eliminate these experiences (and the associated belief that such experiences are problematic and must be corrected). In essence, self-focused attention requires the problematic belief that one's negative thoughts or feelings must be attended to at the exclusion of more relevant stimuli. Of course, basic to the MAC model is the premise that the human experience will involve a multitude of random thoughts and feelings that can be noticed, observed, and passively allowed to pass as we maintain focus on the relevant task at hand.

SESSION REVIEW AND BRIEF CENTERING EXERCISE

As the session draws to an end, it is time to review the forms that the client has completed. This week, as always, the client was asked to complete the What I Have Learned Form as well as the Committing to Performance Values Exercise introduced during this module. The consultant may ask the client to again complete the Emotion and Performance Interference Form used during Module 4 if the client has yet to fully understand the degree to which and the ways in which emotions direct the client's behavior. The choice of asking or not asking for this or any form to be completed is always based on the consultant's judgment. But we suggest that being conservative and going slow rarely leads to poor outcomes. On the other hand, hasty movement from one module to the next and failure to readdress previous topic areas to endure comprehension can certainly delay progress. As always, the session ends with a Brief Centering Exercise intended to refocus and energize the client for his or her next daily activity.

COMMON PROBLEMS SEEN IN MODULE 5

There are two primary difficulties that emerge during Module 5. The first involves difficulties discerning values, goals, potential barriers, and specific performance-related behaviors that need to be activated. The second involves difficulties in moving forward with performance-relevant mindfulness activities.

Values, Goals, Potential Barriers, and Specific Performance-Related Behaviors

As was the case in Module 3, when values and values-directed behavior were introduced, the first difficulty that the client can expect to face in Module 5 is confusion between values and goals. It can be helpful here to again discuss the difference between values as reflecting the *journey* one experiences in the pursuit of achievements, and goals as reflecting the *outcome* associated with one's efforts. Both are important, and they are certainly connected, but they are also very different. Personal performance values can best be described as how you want to remember the day-to-day experiences and approach to your performance life, and how you want others to remember you. On the other hand, goals can best be described as the performance-related achievements, both personal and team, that matter most to you. It should be clear to the consultant and communicated to the client that, when individuals act in the service of their values in a consistent and committed manner, the chances of achieving their goals are substantially greater.

There are times when clients cannot easily describe their values. In these cases, efforts at identifying values lead to statements that are more appropriately defined as goals. We discussed this issue previously in Module 3, but it is fairly common that individuals who experienced earlier problems with this issue will again manifest these difficulties. When faced with this difficulty, the consultant should patiently engage in a dialogue that allows for an appropriate understanding of the distinction between values and goals. With some patient persistence, this issue can be overcome. It is especially helpful to use the Committing to Performance Values Exercise contained in this module to help discriminate values and goals. Through the use of this exercise, the client can gain a clearer understanding of the distinction between values and goals and will be well on the way to isolating the specific behaviors that need to be activated in the service of his or her performance values.

It is important for the consultant to take the time needed to carefully connect the relationship between fundamental values, short- and long-term goals (typically achievement goals), and specific behaviors that will need to be activated on a regular and consistent basis to achieve those values and goals. The careful explication of these behaviors is important and should be achieved collaboratively with the client. It is crucial that the behaviors identified are relevant to the goals and values identified, are within the client's control (do not require the permission or decision of another person), and are truly likely to be reinforced if exhibited. For example, the client who identifies being assertive with teammates as a component of his or her commitment to taking on more of a leadership role in the team/organization may or may not be reinforced for this behavior based on his or her position on the team, tenure with the team, and previous history. The consultant can help the client select the behaviors in the service of his or her values that are most likely to be reinforced and thus result in positive outcomes. Of course, the consultant must fully understand the ways in which activating relevant behaviors in the service of goals and values works to enhance performance. When performance-relevant behaviors are increased in frequency and intensity, skill sets are likely to be better developed and both self- and social reinforcement are likely to be increased. This reinforcement increases the likelihood that the performance-relevant behaviors will continue to be exhibited (likely at an even greater frequency), which further enhances skill sets and overt performance. The belief is that the behaviors to be exhibited will be relevant to skill development and that both self- and social reinforcement will follow. Failure to carefully consider the systemic context of the client's desired behavior change may result in negative outcomes, usually due to either the absence of social reinforcement or, worse, the presence of aversive consequences. In turn, this will inevitably result in the reduction of these performance-relevant behaviors and possibly the complete rejection of the consultant and his or her efforts. As such, the consultant should carefully consider the performance relevance of the specific behaviors that have been identified as related to performance goals and values. A careful consideration of the likely social consequences of these efforts also should be undertaken.

Another, less frequent, problem arises when the *consultant* does not understand the distinction between values and goals or, worse, overtly states to the client that values and goals are essentially the same. Although this is a rare occurrence, it is most likely to be seen when individuals who are not committed to nor versed in the acceptance model are asked or expected to use the MAC program. We cannot stress strongly enough the need to fully understand and commit to this program before engaging in its use. We have seen frustration among both clients and consultants when individuals who are either unsure about or are personally disconnected from the basic theoretical model inappropriately utilize acceptance-based approaches like MAC.

Problems in Moving Forward With Performance-Relevant Mindfulness Activities

As discussed in Module 4, the second half of the MAC protocol requires ongoing and consistent utilization of mindfulness practice, not only during private activity at home, but also in the context of increasingly complex performance-related activities. Initially, we began activity-based mindfulness with an exercise such as washing a dish, moved to mindfulness of natural daily activities such as walking and eating, and then moved to mindfulness of basic physical acts such as stretching and other basic drills and activities. At this point, it is necessary to move the client forward to mindful performance of even more complex skills. Because these can take many forms, the consultant should collaboratively and creatively work with the client to select manageable and relevant activities. While the use of mindfulness while performing is the ultimate goal, it is achieved by increasing use of mindfulness across varying situations instead of through direct assignment. The goal is to help the client develop his or her capacity to be present and aware, in a nonjudging way, across a number of performance-related activities. This can include doing the BCE during natural breaks in competition or work to refocus and decenter from one's thoughts and emotions. As previously noted, it must be understood that the ongoing use and expansion of mindfulness is the foundation on which the rest of the MAC protocol is based. Although somewhat less time is spent on mindfulness practice and discussion in later sessions, it can never be seen as anything less than of the highest importance to the entire MAC protocol.

MODULE 5 CONSIDERATIONS FOR WORKING WITH CLIENTS EXPERIENCING PERFORMANCE DYSFUNCTION

The most difficult aspect of Module 5 when working with clients experiencing performance dysfunction is the behavioral rigidity that often characterizes Pdy. Whether extreme perfectionism, subclinical levels of worry, or dysfunctional relationship patterns are interfering with optimal performance, a common core psychological process is behavioral rigidity.

In this context, behavioral rigidity can be defined in behavioral terms as stimulus generalization in which different situations are responded to in the same or a similar manner. This is best described as repetitive behavior that continues even when there is evidence that the behavior is not working in the individual's best interest. In fact, it easily could be argued that this rigidity is exactly what creates both performance dysfunction and performance impairment, as noted in chapter 3. Conversely, it logically follows that, since behavioral rigidity is a core aspect of the dysfunction, the development of more flexible behavior is necessary for improved performance and better personal functioning.

For individuals with performance dysfunction, the development of a linkage between values, goals, and behavior might not result in behavior change as easily as one would anticipate. For clients with an identifiable performance dysfunction, the activation of new behaviors may be remarkably difficult. Not only do these clients typically manifest behavioral rigidity, but they also tend to find it very hard to break away from their personal rules about the value of worry and rumination, the intolerability of emotion, and so on. Although we do not necessarily suggest that the MAC approach be abandoned for these individuals, we do suggest that the consultant allocate greater time and attention to small incremental behavioral activation. In addition, it is even more important for the consultant to connect the concepts of acceptance and willingness, because ultimately relevant performance behaviors will be activated in clients experiencing performance dysfunction only if they develop the willingness to have their internal experiences (even those that are uncomfortable), decenter from these experiences, and still engage in the necessary behaviors for both goal achievement and the pursuit of their performance values. The consultant may have to again dissuade the client from the assumption that behavior must *follow* mood. Frequently, when working with clients whose performance dysfunction is due to strongly held internal rules (or schemas) about such issues as the meaning of emotions, relationships, adequate and inadequate treatment by those in authority, and so on, it becomes necessary to patiently go back to the concept that internal experiences such as thoughts or emotions are not the explanation for or the cause of one's behavior. While the idea that internal experiences are the reason for one's actions is highly prevalent, particularly in Western cultures, the consultant should again guide the client to a new relationship with his or her internal experience. This, of course, brings us back to the idea that *values* should be the direct cause of one's behavior instead of the thoughts or emotions that are present in any given moment.

It is not uncommon for clients who had little difficulty with the idea of acceptance to demonstrate a brief increase in experiential avoidance as they begin to try out, or even contemplate activating, valued behavior. This is because clients often have a sophisticated intellectual understanding of the concept of acceptance and are therefore "on board" during sessions. However, when the consultant asks the client to take it to the next level by actually *acting* in a more accepting manner, the client realizes that it is not as easy or pleasant as he or she may have believed. As such, clients may experience *more* avoidance for a brief time, based on these new feelings. The consultant should not view this as a setback, should normalize this experience to the client, and should encourage clients to take their negative feelings with them as they engage in valued actions. Revisiting the previous aspects of the model may be initiated as needed.

The following vignette illustrates a client who has been self-referred for performance enhancement in her chosen field of fiction writing. The vignette highlights an apparent problem in activating behavioral change and the need to effectively utilize previously learned concepts of acceptance and willingness to promote performance-relevant behavioral activation:

CONSULTANT: Joan, I can tell by the expression on your face that you are uneasy with the idea that you can act in the manner that we just outlined in the Committing to Performance Values exercise. Are you a little uncomfortable?

CLIENT: I don't know. Maybe a little.

CONSULTANT: What are you uncomfortable with?

CLIENT: I know what we just did looks good on paper, but I know myself. I will sit down to put in 3 hours of work. You know, to continue to write my book in the morning, but I will start thinking, "What's the use, no one will want this, it will just get rejected anyway," and then I will immediately start feeling like crap. Once that happens, I'll get up and find something else to do until I feel better.

CONSULTANT: You mentioned that earlier, while we were working on the form, so you are obviously concerned about it, but what will keep you from doing the 3 hours of work regardless of what you think and feel?

CLIENT: I just can't imagine doing this until I can really believe in myself.

CONSULTANT: Sounds to me like you are totally believing what your mind is telling you, rather than viewing this internal dialogue as just something that happens, something that you learned to do a long time ago. How does your mindfulness practice relate to these thoughts and feelings?

CLIENT: I guess I really do believe it. The mindfulness? Well, if I had those thoughts during mindfulness, sometimes I would go with them, and sometimes I would just let them go and refocus on my breathing.

CONSULTANT: Can you see yourself doing a mindfulness exercise before, in the middle, and toward the end of your 3 hours . . . or even whenever needed, as an aid to just have and not judge the thoughts and emotions, to see them as neither good nor bad, right nor wrong? You see, remember that you don't have to make them go away. As we discussed a few weeks ago, you may, in fact, have these thoughts forever. But, if you can develop the ability to see them as just thoughts and not necessarily forcing your actions, which is how you described them to me a few minutes ago, maybe they can exert less control over your choices.

CLIENT: I guess I can use this as a performance-related mindfulness exercise, like we talked about earlier. It just seems so hard. I am sure other people don't need to work this hard to do their jobs.

CONSULTANT: I'm not sure about that. We all have to learn to perform when we have all sorts of thoughts and emotions. The key is to have them, notice them, let go of them, and refocus on the task. And, maybe most importantly, be willing to feel bad *and* perform well. You are working at letting go of the idea that you want to perform well *but* you feel bad. That is a central component of what we are trying to help you with here. So, you will integrate the mindfulness into this process?

CLIENT: Yes. I really do want to finish this project, it means a great deal to me.

CONSULTANT: I know that, but maybe even more important is you being able to look at yourself as engaging in and even enjoying the journey. Remember your values here. The completion of the project is the achievement goal that comes along with this value.

CLIENT: Okay. I think maybe I'm ready.

CONSULTANT: Great. Just use the form each day to record how it goes.

CLIENT: Will do.

In this vignette, the client presents with a strongly held belief that what she thinks is absolute truth, and thus she sees herself as unable to increase her time on task. She clearly presents her desire to avoid the experience of emotion. The consultant again takes her through the concept of cognitive defusion, or reducing the believability of thoughts, and suggests the use of mindfulness as a means to aid in this process. The consultant also points out the normality of performing while feeling bad as opposed to requiring that bad feelings go away in order to function. This vignette also demonstrates the value of the Committing to Performance Values Exercise as a means of helping the client with this issue. Most importantly, this vignette points out the intense struggle that many clients, particularly those experiencing performance dysfunction, have with the concept of accepting—as opposed to eliminating—thoughts and emotions.

CHAPTER 9

MAC Module 6: Skill Consolidation and Poise— Combining Mindfulness, Acceptance, and Commitment

The primary goal of Module 6 is to help the client attain and maintain greater behavioral flexibility. The consultant encourages the continued use of mindfulness (and, in turn, cognitive defusion) to promote an increasing willingness to accept and fully experience the wide range of internal experiences likely to occur in the service of personally meaningful performance values. The consultant looks to expand upon previous sessions by identifying the situations and thoughts and emotions that have been most problematic. It is likely that these situations and their associated internal experiences have been avoided at the expense of behaviors and choices that would facilitate optimal levels of performance. These behaviors and choices may include practicing when stressed or tired, attending meetings when bored or preoccupied, making necessary work-related phone calls, or going to the gym when distressed or frustrated. These are all examples of situations that are systematically avoided due to some uncomfortable internal state. Thus, the focus of this module is to again present the concept of poise, which was defined as the capacity to act in one's own best interest and function in the service of performance values *regardless* of thoughts and emotions. To enhance the client's poise, the consultant helps the client identify various situations and emotions that have been personally problematic (the source of avoidance) and carefully plan to engage in behaviors that are *opposite* to the avoidant behaviors exhibited. For example, consider the salesperson who avoids setting up necessary meetings with her manager because the manager's style of behavior typically includes the use of criticism. The consultant would encourage the client to go out of her way to set up the meeting. Likewise, if an athlete reports a tendency to avoid or take short cuts at the gym in his off-season training, the consultant could encourage a weekly plan that places the client in the gym for an even greater period of time than might be required. These are called opposite-action plans (Linehan, 1993). While setting up opposite-action plans, the consultant helps the client recognize that they will be uncomfortable performing these tasks. Consistent with the MAC model, the goal of these tasks is *not* reduction of discomfort, but rather the development of the capacity to feel bad and still do what is necessary to perform optimally.

The consultant again includes in-session mindfulness practice during Module 6 and should continue to encourage between-session mindfulness practice, including the extension of performance-relevant mindfulness activities. In addition, during this module, task-focused attention training is added as an extension of mindfulness practice for the purpose of further developing a task-focused attentional style in the pursuit of enhanced performance. As is always the case, the consultant should carefully review material covered in previous modules and review between-session exercises prior to initiating new exercises or introducing new concepts.

Outline of Module 6

1. In-Session Mindfulness Exercises
2. Review of Previous Session
3. Putting It All Together: Enhancing Poise Through Exposure-Based Activities
4. Review and Assign Performance-Relevant Mindfulness and Task-Focused Attention Exercises
5. Brief Centering Exercise and Review of Between-Session Forms

IN-SESSION MINDFULNESS EXERCISES

This module begins with the Brief Centering Exercise to reinforce the commitment to and focus on regular mindfulness practice as a core MAC skill. This exercise allows the client to focus attention in the moment and thus maximizes the client's ability to become fully involved in the session. Of course, this is also an opportunity to ensure that the client has continued to regularly practice mindfulness and presents an additional opportunity for the consultant to discuss experiences that the client has had with regular mindfulness practice. It is also an optimal time to follow up on any issues or problems that may be occurring in the context of regular mindfulness practice.

Following the BCE, the consultant introduces the client to the Task-Focused Attention Exercise. This exercise is introduced to the client as an exercise that will help develop the capacity to redirect attention away from the self and onto the relevant external task at hand. We suggest that the consultant use this opportunity to again briefly discuss the deleterious impact that self-focused attention has on performance (as discussed in chapter 1). The Task-Focused Attention Exercise is similar to previous mindfulness exercises in that awareness of the direction of attention is enhanced, and the capacity to focus fully on all aspects of a situation is optimized. Yet this exercise differs from previous mindfulness exercises in that it is intended to promote attentional redirection *during* the most difficult situations, rather than hoping that the redirection of attention learned in other mindfulness exercises will generalize to difficult situations. In the exercise, which is described below, the client is asked to focus attention on a contrived task under increasingly difficult circumstances. The exercise moves from attention-to-task with no stressful stimuli present to a scenario involving greater interpersonal stress and, finally, to one that requires the ability to focus on an external task in the face of stress.

Task-Focused Attention Exercise

This brief exercise will help develop the capacity to redirect attention from internal experiences such as thoughts (i.e., "how am I doing?") and feelings (such as anxiety) to the performance task at hand. After completing the BCE, the client and consultant sit so that the client's back is to the consultant, and no eye contact can occur. The consultant then relays a 2-minute story about a recent event in his or her life. The client is instructed to concentrate on the story. When the story is complete, the client is asked to recount the story in as much detail as possible, after which the consultant asks the client to talk about what other stimuli, either internal (thoughts) or external (noises) the client was aware of.

This portion of the exercise is repeated using a different story each time until the client can recount a significant amount of the story's details (well more than 50%). Once the client can successfully complete this portion of the exercise, the client is asked to face the consultant and listen to another story. This time, the consultant and client are to hold eye contact during the entire story. Once again, the client is asked to recount story details following completion of the story. This portion of the exercise is also repeated until well more than 50% of the story's details can be recounted. Each repeated presentation requires a new story.

Finally, in the last portion of this exercise, the client should describe a recent past or upcoming stressful performance-related event in some detail (the consultant should ask questions and promote images that are likely to enhance the experience of negative affect). Immediately following the promotion of negative affect, the consultant should present a new 2-minute story, with the client again having to recount details upon completion. This procedure is repeated until well more than 50% of the story's details are recounted.

It is important to remember that the goal of this exercise is not the reduction of anxiety. Many clients will describe increasing levels of discomfort as the exercise moves forward. The goals of the exercise are twofold. The first goal is to help the client develop the capacity to gently move his or her focus of attention from internal processes such as emotions, thoughts, and bodily sensations (self-focused attention) to more task-appropriate external stimuli (story details verbalized by the consultant). Second, in the course of completing this exercise, the client can see that, even with anxiety or frustration, he or she can focus attention as needed for the task at hand. For many clients, this will be a clear and observable opportunity to experience what has been presented throughout the entire MAC program—clients can experience uncomfortable emotion and still function (in this case attend) as needed, and this can be done with absolutely no need to minimize, eliminate, or otherwise control their emotional states.

Upon completion of the exercise, the consultant should discuss the experience with the client. This exercise is typically quite illuminating and results in interesting conversation about attention and the ability to function even when faced with extraneous thoughts and emotions. For many clients, this exercise is also empowering, in that it may be one of the first times that the client has "let go" of his or her self-focused attention. Thus, the exercise may be viewed as an experience that enhances one's personal self-efficacy regarding the ability to truly accomplish both the objectives of the MAC program and one's personal goals.

REVIEW OF PREVIOUS SESSION

After the BCE and Task-Focused Attention Exercise is a discussion of the material covered in the previous session, possibly by using the What I Have Learned Form (see chapter 4) if the consultant has continued to use this form. This represents an opportunity for the consultant to respond to questions, monitor progress, and provide feedback as needed. This is particularly important at this juncture of the MAC program, because the last module began the process of activating behaviors that were identified as being in the best interest of the client's performance values, and, as such, it can be expected that a great deal of emotion and possibly avoidance has emerged. However, the client may not overtly report increased emotion and avoidance. Clients may instead state a lack of understanding of the previous week's material, when what is really occurring is an effort to explain away avoidance. The consultant should, therefore, carefully consider whether expressions of uncertainty truly reflect uncertainty and should watch for subtle, in-session (socially acceptable) manifestation of experiential avoidance.

During this portion of Module 6, the consultant will also carefully review and discuss in detail the Committing to Performance Values Exercise. Successes with the exercise should be strongly reinforced, and difficulties in completing the form or in engaging in the specific behaviors highlighted during the previous session must be understood and discussed. It is imperative that difficulties with this exercise and with between-session activation of performance-relevant behaviors be addressed before moving on to any additional information. As noted throughout the protocol, it is better to take all the time necessary to ensure that the client both understands the material and has begun to integrate the concepts into his or her life before moving forward to new material or concepts. This may require one or more modules to be completed over multiple sessions. If the client has had serious difficulty in completing recent tasks, or if the client has not engaged in the tasks (including completion of the Committing to Performance Values Exercise), we suggest returning to the appropriate component of the previous module before progressing to the core goals of Module 6. This could be necessary for any client type and, as discussed later in this chapter, will often be necessary for clients experiencing performance dysfunction.

PUTTING IT ALL TOGETHER: ENHANCING POISE THROUGH EXPOSURE-BASED ACTIVITIES

Enhancing poise is the core goal of Module 6 and requires the client to effectively use his or her developing skills relating to mindfulness, acceptance, and commitment. This segment of Module 6 begins with a thorough review and discussion of the Committing to Performance Values Exercise completed by the client during the previous week. The exercise should be thoroughly reviewed and discussed, the client should be reinforced for his or her efforts, and failure to activate behaviors that were defined during the previous module should be carefully reviewed. The consultant will gently yet directly confront avoidance and the consequences that inevitably follow, while validating the reality that, for some individuals, long-held avoidance patterns can be difficult to break. It is often at this point in the MAC program that the consultant will notice in-session behaviors that suggest a reduction of avoidance. A prime example of this is more direct and rapid "owning up" to avoidance behavior. By this point, some clients will immediately acknowledge that they chose the easy way by not activating their behavior during the previous week. When this occurs, the consultant and client may confront a different type of difficult situation. Namely, sharing the truth with the consultant risks the consultant's disapproval and disappointment. When the client begins to acknowledge his or her avoidance more rapidly, it is beneficial to immediately point it out and reinforce it. In doing so, the consultant can use this in-session behavior change as a springboard for more difficult between-session behavior change. In our experience, over half of clients do not fully complete the Committing to Performance Values Exercise the first time assigned, and persistence on the part of the consultant is necessary to move forward. This is especially true for clients experiencing any form of performance dysfunction.

When the client has successfully completed the Committing to Performance Values Exercise, the consultant can begin to focus on performance-specific behaviors in need of activation by helping the client confront—and function in the face of—specific situations that have been most problematic and emotionally evocative in the past. The first targets of behavioral activation should certainly be relevant, yet should not be too difficult or important in the pursuit of enhanced performance. Remember that the overarching MAC goal at this point is to help clients perform in the face of difficult situations and emotions. This is achieved by encouraging and structuring behavioral activities that will place the client into situations that have been difficult or problematic in the past. The client will then be instructed to engage in affirmative (approach) behaviors that are likely to be performance enhancing, rather than the performance-negating avoidance behaviors that the client has used in the past. Through the process of habituation, it is likely that the client will experience a reduction of distress while going through these guided experiences. However, the reduction of negative thoughts or emotions is secondary and should not be emphasized in discussions with the client. Although the client may appreciate such distress reduction, it is not the goal of the MAC program or other acceptance-based models. The focus is on development of a willingness to experience negative thoughts and emotions in the service of performance-relevant values. For consultants trained in the behavioral tradition, encouraging clients to confront and function despite their distress will be a familiar concept. The clinical use of these experiences is often referred to as "exposure," which is a core process for the alleviation of numerous behavioral difficulties (Barlow, 2001).

As previously described, the term *poise* denotes the ability to experience distress and still function as needed. In our experience, performers view this term positively and can comprehend the benefits of developing this skill. Developing or enhancing poise requires the client to systematically confront difficult emotionally charged situations and act in a manner that is often the complete opposite of how they previously responded—that is, approach rather than avoid. As such, the client will engage in actions that promote performance values rather than engaging in actions that achieve short-term relief from distress.

To effectively utilize this opposite-action behavioral approach to difficult situations, it is essential that the consultant and client first identify the performance-related situations that are most difficult to deal with and then develop a proactive—as opposed to reactive—strategy for dealing with the situation. For example, we recently worked with a high-level business executive whose job required him to make significant cuts in expenditures. These cuts would impact a number of long-term employees, many of whom had become friends of his over the years. His personal behavioral style was one that utilized experiential avoidance to reduce the likelihood that significant people in his life would become angry with him, and, consistent with this approach, he avoided making many of these essential cuts out of a desire to avoid the interpersonal consequence (having to face the unhappiness and distress of others). His boss was becoming increasingly frustrated with his lack of attention to this corporate mandate, and our client began to experience even higher levels of stress. His approach had been a *reactive* one in which he would act only when he had to, and, in doing so, he behaved less effectively as an executive. Working together, we developed a hierarchy of situations that would require the client to proactively contact a number of employees and give them negative news (feedback, corporate mandates, etc.), beginning with those employees who he predicted would respond least poorly. The hierarchy culminated in contacting the individuals who he predicted would respond most negatively to the information. The client was asked to complete the task over the course of the next week.

The following vignette is taken from work with this client and demonstrates how the consultant can seamlessly move from the Committing to Performance Values Exercise to the point of defining the hierarchy of difficult situations for the following week.

CONSULTANT: Let's take a look at how you did with the Committing to Performance Values Exercise since our last session.

CLIENT: I think it went pretty well. I wrote it all down . . . here it is (hands over form). You remember that we identified my being seen as a reliable boss as my performance value. We identified the short-term goal as getting better performance from my sales staff, and the long-term goal was my own standing in the company, and that my own personal compensation would increase as a result. The behavior that we identified we would need to rev up was responding more immediately to my staff when they needed me, even if that meant more work for me. You can see here (points to form) that the situation I wrote down was a day that I had three calls from senior sales staff, all needing all kinds of information from me. My first thought was to call maybe one and leave the rest until the next day, but I realized what my mind was telling me and decided to make all the calls.

CONSULTANT: What was the barrier that you faced?

CLIENT: It took a long time to gather up the information they needed, and I was really stressed out the entire day. But I did end up getting the information and called each one. I think they were shocked! (Laughs) So here (points to form), I would rate this activity as a 10 because I think it really contributed to my work performance.

CONSULTANT: I think that is really outstanding. You really did a great job. Would you say this is one of the most difficult performance-related issues that you could have faced?

CLIENT: I wish it was, but really, having to give bad news is much more difficult for me. I think I have this thing about needing to be liked and when I have to tell people bad news, especially people that I care about, I feel really bad.

CONSULTANT: Actually, feeling bad when you give people you care about bad news sounds pretty normal to me. I would call that a *clean* emotion, one that the vast majority of people have, and one that is very appropriate. After all, do you really want to be someone who doesn't care about the feelings of others?

CLIENT: Oh, absolutely not. So you're saying it's okay when I get uncomfortable with something like this?

CONSULTANT: Of course it's okay. But you're saying much more, I think. It sounds to me like you're saying that if you feel badly about giving someone bad news, you try to avoid doing it so you avoid feeling bad.

CLIENT: Yes, exactly. I'll give you an example. I have a corporate mandate to cut costs. This means telling senior sales staff, some people I've known for years and am pretty close with, that they have to reduce their expense accounts. What's worse is that, in some cases, even their guaranteed salaries may be reduced! I just feel like I can't do it. So, I've been avoiding it over and over . . . to the point that my own boss is getting angry. I feel like it's crazy, because I'm risking my own standing in the company because I can't deal with people being upset at me.

CONSULTANT: So, the issue is not how you feel, but the choices that you make. It sounds like the choice you have made is to put not feeling bad ahead of doing your job and being known as a reliable executive.

CLIENT: This is going to be really difficult for me.

CONSULTANT: Well . . . then that's where we go now. Let's put together a list, from easiest to hardest, of the people you need to give some bad news to, and set up a plan to go out and get it done, no matter how you feel, this coming week.

CLIENT: Awww, I was afraid you were going to say that. (Laughs) Okay, I know we need to work on this.

This vignette begins by taking the client through a review of the Committing to Performance Values Exercise. It progresses through the identification of the next course of action, opposite-action behavior. This will, by definition, involve *prolonged exposure* to the difficult emotions that have typified these situations in the past. The client is now ready to take his commitment to activating behaviors in the service of his goals and values to the next level. He will be confronting the most difficult and often avoided situations. This serves the ultimate purpose of the entire MAC program, which is to increase the client's engagement in activities that will ultimately make him or her more productive in his or her performance world.

The point of the *Committing to Performance Values Exercise* is to have clients act in a manner that is both effective in the pursuit of their stated performance goals and values, and at the same time act in an opposite manner to the behavioral approach they would normally take.

It should be expected that many clients will require multiple sessions focusing on this exercise. For a couple of additional sessions, the consultant may work with the client to successfully identify other difficult situations that require a more proactive approach. Additional assignments would be developed and assigned as needed.

Successful completion of this assignment requires the integration of the MAC skills taught to date: (a) attention to the task at hand; (b) awareness of one's internal processes, with an associated willingness to experience these reactions; and (c) activating oneself to engage in actions that serve performance-related goals and values instead of actions that lead to short-term reduction of distress. This assignment promotes choosing to perform necessary proactive behaviors in the face of, and despite, discomfort. This is ultimately our definition of poise!

REVIEW AND ASSIGN PERFORMANCE-RELEVANT MINDFULNESS AND TASK-FOCUSED ATTENTION EXERCISES

In Module 6, the consultant continues to help the client move closer to mindful engagement in competition by ensuring that mindfulness practice becomes increasingly utilized in performance-related situations. Each session should involve a discussion of performance-related mindfulness activities performed during the previous week. During each session, the performance-relevant mindfulness activities that were practiced during the previous week should be explored for frequency, length of time, outcome of use, problems or surprises associated with use, and, finally, a discussion about extending these activities into new situations for the following week.

At this point in the MAC program, it is appropriate for the consultant to suggest that a performance-relevant version of the Task-Focused Attention Exercise be practiced between sessions. For example, keeping with how the exercise was practiced earlier in Module 6, the consultant might suggest that, during the next week, the performer listen to a coach's or manager's instructions in the same manner that he or she listened to the consultant in the previous session. The following week, the client will describe the amount of material remembered immediately following the coach's/manager's talk. Or, the performer may choose to take a moment during which he or she is watching someone else perform (i.e., while on the bench or in a meeting) and notice as many details as possible. The client should be instructed to note which details he or she attended to and the frequency of random thoughts, and then repeat the procedure again and again until the amount of detail attended to increases substantially (as in the original in-session exercise).

The consultant should make it clear that the purpose of these exercises is to enhance attention and concentration, not by eliminating random thoughts and emotions, but despite thoughts and emotions. Random internal experiences are natural and will inevitably occur. The goal is to allow these events to occur without dominating one's attentional processes.

BRIEF CENTERING EXERCISE AND REVIEW OF
BETWEEN-SESSION FORMS

As with other sessions, this session should end with a review of the forms that the client has been asked to complete. This week, the consultant may again ask the client to complete the What I Have Learned Form as well as the Committing to Performance Values Exercise. The latter is essential in promoting and monitoring the client's new efforts at behavioral activation. In particular, it can be used to monitor the client's efforts at opposite-action behavior.

The material and exercises covered in Module 6 are surely challenging, but are a giant step toward optimal performance. We suggest that moving more slowly through certain parts of the MAC program may lead to better outcomes for some clientele. The consultant should not assume that a commitment to performance values is intact without a tangible demonstration of this commitment. This may best be seen through the activation of defined behaviors. For some clients, this process will take hold immediately and gather speed as it is naturally reinforced by immediate performance improvements and social consequences. Yet with other clients, especially those with entrenched patterns of experiential avoidance, the activation of values-directed behaviors will be more difficult and will take considerably more time and patience to achieve.

As always, the session ends with the Brief Centering Exercise intended to refocus and energize the client for his or her next daily activity.

COMMON PROBLEMS SEEN IN MODULE 6

The most common problems associated with Module 6 center on the client's willingness or unwillingness to change behavior. Most clients who seek psychological intervention would like to have the outcomes they desire. Most individuals who seek relationship counseling would like a better relationship. Finally, most people who are anxious or depressed certainly seek psychological treatment with a desire to feel better. The problem is that many people want these outcomes without having to make significant changes in the way they behave. They would like change to occur, yet in many cases they desire for this to be somewhat of a magical experience. The therapist, counselor, or consultant is expected to provide some magical answer or some formula for life to be better without requiring the client to engage in any real behavior change. Perhaps most individuals would deny that this is the case. Yet anyone who has spent more than 10 minutes with clients will certainly recognize that many clients do not understand the degree to which their own behaviors are at the center of their difficulties. In fact, behavioral rigidity, which refers to doing the same thing over and over again despite its obvious ineffectiveness, is the hallmark of psychological disturbance. Individuals in dysfunctional relationships often do not fully comprehend the degree to which their behaviors contribute to the problems. Anxious and depressed individuals may not fully understand the degree to which avoidance and behavioral deactivation contribute to their difficulties. Similarly, performers who want to perform better sometimes fail to recognize that their fundamental approach to their performance lives directly contributes to their lack of consistent or enhanced performance. This point in the MAC protocol requires clear behavioral change, often requiring behavior that is completely opposite of what the client has done before (and thus overlearned). Given these requirements, some clients will find this part of the MAC program very difficult. Yet this is precisely why it works. The breaking of avoidance behaviors frees the client to be more flexible, and the client can more effectively respond to his or her performance world.

Not surprisingly, some clients will not complete the behavior change assignments given in Modules 5 and 6. This will often be noted first when the client has not completed the Committing to Performance Values Exercise. Such clients typically state one of two reasons for their lack of behavior change efforts: "I didn't really understand" and "There wasn't an opportunity to do this stuff this week." However, if the consultant provided enough time for a thorough discussion of this activity, understanding should not be an issue. This possible explanation should still be explored, and, if found to be true, the consultant should go back to the beginning of Module 5 rather than trying to move along to Module 6. On the other hand, if it becomes apparent that lack of effort is the reason for the incomplete activity (which is more likely to be the case), a discussion relating to values becomes critical. Here, the consultant should pay special attention to whether the underlying issue is a lack of commitment or another example of experiential avoidance. Although most clients recognize that behavioral activation is an important step toward optimal performance, behavioral activation will almost certainly be uncomfortable for the client to some extent. It should be discussed early that the client *will* experience some discomfort and may therefore even doubt the value of the activity. This is so common because most of us have learned that whatever makes us feel bad should be eliminated. Thus, if the client has acted to avoid discomfort at the expense of behavioral change in the service of his or her stated values, a review and discussion of this core MAC concept should be repeated.

We encourage consultants to remember that avoidance of behavior change is not necessarily *resistance* in the traditional sense of the word. Although it may reflect a poorly formed or noncollaborative relationship between the consultant and client, the lack of true desire to work with the consultant, or a lack of confidence in the consultant, it may just as likely be a direct reflection of the precise issue that has been interfering with consistent and optimal performance. Thus, rather than becoming frustrated with the client or seeing the lack of execution of between-session exercises as indicative of a problematic client attitude, we suggest that the consultant view this as a learning opportunity. In essence, when the client fails to complete this or any other between-session exercise, it provides an opportunity to demonstrate to the client the impact of avoidance. This can be witnessed at that very moment, right in the midst of the session. The most significant new learning opportunities for clients often come during these difficult and frustrating within-session moments.

The following vignette describes this new learning opportunity:

CONSULTANT: I see that you didn't complete the Committing to Performance Values Exercise since the last session. What's going on?

CLIENT: There really wasn't any opportunity this week and I was really busy with stuff that had to get done.

CONSULTANT: Tell me a little bit about the stuff that had to get done.

CLIENT: Just a lot of life stuff.

CONSULTANT: I can understand that. So, tell me about times you thought about completing the form and decided to complete it at another time.

CLIENT: Well . . . When I did think about it, there was always something else that needed to be done and I just didn't want to deal with it.

CONSULTANT: Okay, but I'm a little confused. We talked in previous weeks about how much improving your game means to you, but now it seems like a lot of things were deemed more important. Now, maybe they were . . . but maybe they weren't also, and you put off completing the form because it was in some way uncomfortable and you really didn't want to deal with it. What do you think?

CLIENT: I didn't want to deal with it then, and I don't really want to deal with it now, just like I don't want to deal with a lot of things relating to golf sometimes.

CONSULTANT: All right. That is fine, as long as you realize that you are making this choice. You are avoiding things that are difficult in the service of immediate comfort . . . feeling better, rather than dealing with uncomfortable things that are in the service of the values that *you* identified as being meaningful.

CLIENT: Well, um . . . whatever.

CONSULTANT: It's actually sounding right now like you want to avoid the discomfort of this conversation, so you are doing things to push me away. Does this seem at all familiar to you?

CLIENT: (Laughing) Yeah, my coach always tells me that when I don't want to hear something I just shut down and take my mind far away.

CONSULTANT: Exactly! And how exactly does that help you achieve the things you value?

CLIENT: It doesn't. It just makes my life more difficult.

CONSULTANT: Well. That is true, but you do get something from it. You get to escape from things that make you uncomfortable for a few minutes. The question is, and it goes back to work we have done together earlier in our sessions, is it worth the sacrifice?

CLIENT: No. You're right. Sometimes I'm just kind of a child, I guess.

CONSULTANT: I'm not sure how saying that about yourself helps. Although in some cases, beating yourself up like that might get people to let go of the uncomfortable topic of conversation and give you a break. But, let's keep our eye on the ball, because I think you are stronger than that. Avoidance says *nothing* about your character. It is just a behavioral pattern that you have. You've developed a desire to avoid discomfort even if it is not in your long-term best interest. This is a behavioral style that we have to be vigilant about and work against whenever possible.

This case vignette illustrates avoidance, both in terms of the client's noncompletion of the between-session exercise and the in-session avoidance noted in the style of interaction with the consultant. The consultant not only pointed out the avoidant in-session behavior being manifested by the client, but also connected it to the issue of the between-session assignment and previous difficulties the client has had in getting the maximum benefit from his coaching.

The consultant should remember that avoidance can be seen in both obvious and subtle forms. It is imperative that when the client's avoidant behavior is noted directly in a session, it be gently confronted to help the client move from an avoidance-focused to an approach-focused style of life.

One last potential problem in Module 6 should be considered. People generally do not like feeling uncomfortable, so when presenting the rationale for engaging in exposure-based activities, it is critical for the consultant to point out that the purpose of such activities is to learn to tolerate and experience discomfort—not for its own sake, but to enhance the likelihood that it will lead to optimal performance and sound decision making. The consultant should, therefore, constantly refer back to the concept of developing poise and its connection with optimal performance.

MODULE 6 CONSIDERATIONS FOR WORKING WITH CLIENTS EXPERIENCING PERFORMANCE DYSFUNCTION

Individuals experiencing performance dysfunction are likely to be particularly challenging in the course of completing Module 6. The reason for this speaks to the essence of performance dysfunction. Individuals manifesting Pdy, by the very nature of their difficulties, are likely to find it very difficult to remain task-focused and engage in approach rather than avoidance behavior. By definition, performance dysfunction involves difficulties with emotion regulation. These difficulties manifest as overt behavioral avoidance or as less visible experiential avoidance, characterized by brooding, rumination, and/or worry. These cognitive events, as discussed earlier in this text, serve the function of *cognitive* avoidance, are overlearned (usually in early childhood), and are highly resistant to change.

This being said, Module 6's emphasis on task concentration and poise through experiential acceptance can be effective but can be expected to require a number of sessions. Each session will essentially repeat topics and activities and seek to shape and develop the skills of task concentration and experiential acceptance over a longer period of time than would be expected with non-Pdy clients. We encourage consultants to patiently persist in their efforts and break the basic goals and sections of MAC Module 6 into several units. For example, the section on task-focused attention could easily require two or three sessions, followed by an additional two or three sessions focusing on exposure-based activities. Of course, regular and consistent mindfulness practice is an essential and necessary first step toward the ultimate success of Module 6 with clients experiencing Pdy. If regular and consistent mindfulness practice has not been developed, it is unlikely that Module 6 will be optimally effective. In such cases, initiating Module 6 should be postponed until regular and consistent mindfulness practice is effectively undertaken.

CHAPTER 10

MAC Module 7: Maintaining and Enhancing Mindfulness, Acceptance, and Commitment

By the final MAC module, clients should be regularly engaged in exercises to promote MAC skills that are central to optimal human performance. These skills include:

- *Mindfulness,* to promote enhanced self-awareness and task-focused attention.
- *Acceptance* of uncomfortable thoughts and emotions as a normal part of the human experience. This is noted most clearly as a willingness to experience uncomfortable thoughts and emotions in the service of behaviors that promote and/or attain performance goals and values.
- *Commitment* to behavioral activation through the consistent use of those actions necessary in the pursuit of self-defined performance values.

From this foundation, the primary purpose of this last MAC module is to extend the skills already developed and promote the ongoing use of exercises and behaviors that will allow the performer to maintain and further enhance his or her desired performance following completion of the MAC program.

The first segment of Module 7 is an extension of the Task-Focused Attention Exercise to continue the development of the ability to move attention away from the self and instead place and maintain attention on the demands of the external environment as circumstances dictate. In addition, Module 7 further emphasizes the necessity of continued practice and the development of basic and performance-relevant mindfulness exercises to further develop the capacity to see thoughts and emotions as *simply* thoughts and emotions. Previously referred to as decentering, this ability is very important during both performance and nonperformance life situations.

The second segment of Module 7 reemphasizes the need to be vigilant regarding both obvious and subtle forms of avoidance. By doing so, the performer remains willing to experience the variety of normal discomforts that life inevitably brings. Willingness should occur in the context of continuing to pursue valued performance goals through the activation of necessary behaviors, many of which are likely to be contrary (even opposite) to previously learned behavioral patterns.

The overarching purpose of Module 7 is to prepare the client for the completion of the MAC program by stressing the lifelong nature of these skills and exercises. As such, the third and final segment of Module 7 involves the establishment of a specific plan for the practice of the entire range of MAC skills over the months following completion of the MAC program. This segment includes the development of a system of appropriate self-monitoring as a means by which the client can self-reflect and self-correct as necessary. This final segment of Module 7 should also include a discussion of progress made, any skills still in need of personal development, and means of contacting the consultant for future booster sessions if needed.

Outline of Module 7

1. Review Previous Session and Overall MAC Program
2. Brief Centering Exercise
3. Task-Focused Attention Exercise
4. Review of Current Level of Experiential Acceptance, Willingness, and Commitment to Values
5. Plan for Future Practice: Self-Reflection and Self-Correction

REVIEW PREVIOUS SESSION AND OVERALL MAC PROGRAM

In the first segment of Module 7, the consultant engages in a comprehensive review of the overall MAC program, followed by a specific review of the material covered in Module 6.

When reviewing the entire MAC program, we suggest that the consultant begin with a review of the initial stated purpose for the client's participation in the program, including a discussion of the performance-related issues and goals that existed at the time the MAC program was initiated. With this as a starting point, the consultant should review the identification of performance-relevant values that the client completed and discuss the distinction between behaviors in the service of experiential avoidance and behaviors in the service of valued goals. Once this distinction is discussed using examples drawn from the work done with the client, it is time for a discussion of the specific skills that have been developed through the MAC program. General and specific mindfulness skills, task-focused attention, experiential acceptance/willingness, and behavioral commitment/activation are all skills that the client has systematically worked on over the course of the first six modules of the MAC. It is in the context of this overall discussion of the MAC that the material covered during Module 6 should be carefully reviewed.

At the beginning of Module 7, the consultant should initiate discussion of the client's post-MAC program future. Specifically, the consultant should continue to point out that the skills developed through the course of the MAC program require ongoing time and attention. In this regard, it should be stressed that, by this time, the client has developed skills that are foundational to enhanced performance, and the client can be expected to develop these skills even further with regular practice after the completion of the MAC program.

It is also important that the consultant take some time to discuss the interpersonal aspects related to the impending completion of the MAC program. By this time, it is likely that the client has come to see the consultant as an ally and professional resource. As such, issues relating to the termination of this professional relationship warrant some attention. A combination of reassurance regarding the client's readiness to work on the MAC skills on their own and reassurance that the consultant is only a phone call away if questions or problems arise is usually sufficient to foster an appropriate attitude of independence. We have found that using the metaphor of dental visits often makes the point we wish the client to receive. When you visit a dentist, you may have a prolonged number of visits until the work is done. At that point, while you no longer need regular appointments, it is comforting to know that the dentist is readily available for future needs if they arise. Some individuals will not be able to personally identify with this particular metaphor, so the consultant can tailor the topic to one that would be a good fit for the client. Either way, we suggest that the consultant frame his or her work with the client in a manner that empowers the client to be independent, yet comforted to know that the consultant is available for future help if and when that becomes necessary or desired. Depending on the particular client and any personal issues regarding independence (and possibly abandonment), this discussion may be appropriately handled in one or multiple sessions before completion of the protocol. Special considerations for clients with significant abandonment issues are discussed later in this chapter.

It is important to emphasize that, for clients who have worked hard at developing MAC skills, the end of the formal MAC program may be seen as an end of the MAC experience. It is essential to present that the end of the formal MAC training program is actually only the *beginning*. In essence:

> The end of the MAC program marks the beginning of a lifelong journey of mindful self-awareness, acceptance of the ongoing struggle that life entails, and an ongoing commitment to those actions that are most meaningful to the client, both in and out of the performance world.

Completion of the formal MAC program is in essence a graduation of sorts. We often use a race car metaphor to reiterate this point. Completing the MAC program gives the individual a driver's license. But does it qualify the individual to hit the NASCAR track? It is only through continued hard work and committed action that the individual will fully achieve and maintain optimal performance states. After completing the MAC program, the client is ready to continue the journey through both the performance career and life itself.

BRIEF CENTERING EXERCISE

Module 7 includes the continued in-session use and practice of the Brief Centering Exercise. The use of this exercise all the way through the MAC program, even in this last module, not only continues to demonstrate our commitment to regular mindfulness practice, but also provides the opportunity for the consultant to discuss the development and regular use of mindfulness exercises by the client in the future. Following completion of the BCE, the consultant should evaluate the client's attempt to integrate mindfulness practice into his or her daily routine. This should include regular use of the BCE and/or the Mindfulness of the Breath Exercise practiced earlier in the MAC program. It is important to reinforce regular utilization of mindfulness exercises and again describe the benefits of enhanced mindful awareness and mindful attention, both of which have been discussed in terms of their connection to optimal human performance earlier in the protocol. A brief review of the importance of awareness and attention for all types of human performance may be helpful at this point. Following this review, the consultant will discuss the continued use of performance-relevant mindfulness exercises once the formal portion of the MAC program ends. Up to this point, the consultant has worked with the client to move from practice to pre-event, and eventually to appropriate mid-event performance-relevant mindfulness exercises (i.e., during natural breaks in performance activities). It is critical in this final module for the consultant to make sure that performance-relevant mindfulness activities are being regularly practiced and integrated into the client's performance life. The benefits and any difficulties of integrating mindfulness into the client's performance activities should be thoroughly discussed with an eye toward providing corrective feedback.

We have stressed the need for the consultant to engage in a serious and thoughtful discussion with the client concerning the need for ongoing and regular mindfulness practice following completion of the MAC program. To aid in this endeavor, the consultant is encouraged to develop a formal plan for both regular and performance-relevant mindfulness exercises, which should then be recorded on the Post-MAC Practice Plan Form provided in Figure 10.1.

TASK-FOCUSED ATTENTION EXERCISE

Following the Brief Centering Exercise, the consultant moves to the continuation and further development of task-focused attention through use of the Task-Focused Attention Exercise. As described in Module 6, this exercise will help the client develop the capacity to redirect attention from internal experiences such as thoughts (i.e., "how am I doing?") and feelings (i.e., anxiety) to necessary elements of the actual performance task at hand.

The consultant may find it helpful to begin by reminding the client of the last time he or she performed the exercise, summarizing the results, and discussing the client's previous experiences. This discussion also should include between-session assignments (since the last session) utilizing the exercise.

Once this discussion has been completed and the consultant has reviewed the client's independent efforts to use the Task-Focused Attention Exercise, it is time to engage the client in an effort to enhance task-focused attention in increasingly difficult situations. This process begins with the development of a short hierarchy of difficult, challenging, or threatening performance situations. This hierarchy should be recorded

Post-MAC Practice Plan Form

(Page 1)

Performance Value(s):_____

1. Basic Mindfulness Practice
    a. Exercises to be used
    b. Situations(s) in which it is used
    c. Frequency
    d. Time of day
2. Performance-Relevant Mindfulness Practice
    a. Exercises to be used
    b. Situations(s) in which it is used
    c. Frequency
3. Task-Focused Attention Exercise
    a. Situations(s) in which it is used
    b. Frequency

Record Weekly Mindfulness Practice:

_____

_____

_____

_____

_____

_____

_____

_____

_____

_____

FIGURE 10.1   Post-MAC Practice Plan Form

Post-MAC Practice Plan Form

(Page 2)

4. Acceptance, Willingness, and Commitment
    a. Performance value and associated goal
    b. Obstacle—thoughts and/or emotions
    c. Avoidant behavior(s)
    d. Specific opposite-action behavior(s) to be activated

Record Weekly Behavioral Activation:

_____

_____

_____

_____

_____

_____

_____

_____

_____

_____.

Evaluation of Practice and Use of MAC Skills During the Past Week:

(1 = no use/infrequent use, 5 = moderate use, 10 = frequent use): _____

FIGURE 10.1   Continued.

from easiest to most difficult and should generally include three or four situations (no fewer than two and no more than five). The following steps should be followed when practicing this version of the Task-Focused Attention Exercise, which over time should include increasingly challenging situations:

1. Collect information regarding the following questions:
   a. What is the task and how is successful performance of the task evaluated?
   b. Where has the client's attention most often been focused during these situations in the past?
   c. What are the most relevant external stimuli that require attention during the task?
2. Create the affective experience of the situation through verbal description and imaginal creation of the relevant scene(s).
3. Following intensification of the relevant affect, practice each situation using the basic eye-to-eye Task-Focused Attention Exercise in which the client is instructed to listen to story details and recall the details afterward.
4. Task-focused attention is evaluated in terms of the percentage of story details remembered.
5. The exercise is repeated until well over half of the details can be recounted.
6. Each situation in the hierarchy is systematically utilized as per the directions above.

For some clients, there will be only one or two situations, and the exercise can be performed using both situations in a single session. Other clients (most likely those experiencing performance dysfunction) may have a more extensive hierarchy and will thus require more than one session to complete this portion of the exercise.

Following completion of this entire process, the consultant will review the results and meaning of the exercise and discuss how the client can continue this practice after completion of the formal MAC program. While the client has already practiced this exercise with verbally presented information, he or she also can be encouraged to use visually presented material in future attempts. Inevitably, the client will recall increasing amounts of information, despite feeling increasing levels of anxiety and other forms of affect during the exercise. As this occurs, the consultant can discuss how this demonstrates the fallacy of the belief that negative affect must be reduced in order for someone to remain task-focused. The consultant also may make the point that task-focused attention can be even further increased over time. During this discussion, the consultant and client should record the plan for continued practice of the Task-Focused Attention Exercise on the Post-MAC Practice Plan form.

Consultants should note that we are using the term *formal* MAC program purposefully, because we believe that clients can, and should, remain engaged in an *informal* training and development of the MAC skills long after the formal structured MAC program ends. An apt metaphor for use in this context is the metaphor of personal training for enhanced physical fitness and development. Personal trainers help individuals learn what exercise to use and for what purpose, develop proper exercise technique to maximize their strength and fitness gains, and maintain structure and motivation. In most cases, following some period of formal personal training, individuals begin to train on their own based on what they have previously learned, and they continue their commitment to enhanced physical fitness. In a similar way, we have presented the relationship between the formal consultant-guided MAC program and the less formal, self-guided MAC program that follows. Continued growth and development of the basic MAC skills requires ongoing commitment to self-guided practice. This results in the proper maintenance of program gains for many years to come.

REVIEW OF CURRENT LEVEL OF
EXPERIENTIAL ACCEPTANCE, WILLINGNESS,
AND COMMITMENT TO VALUES

In this segment of Module 7, the consultant reviews the client's performance behaviors (performance preparation as well as work/competition) and evaluates the degree to which experiential acceptance is clearly observable. It is expected at this point that the frequency of experiential acceptance should greatly surpass the frequency of experiential avoidance. The consultant should carefully consider the situations in which experiential avoidance still occurs, especially if it appears to block in some significant way the actions and activities that are central to the performance values of the client. In this context, it is imperative that the consultant works with the client to develop a specific plan to continue his or her effort to overcome this avoidance (see the Post-MAC Practice Plan form). This plan essentially utilizes portions of previous exercises and asks the client to identify: (a) relevant performance values; (b) current obstacles to the active and consistent pursuit of those values; (c) any uncomfortable internal experiences such as thoughts (such as "I can't do this") or emotions (such as anxiety or frustration); (d) behaviors that reflect avoidance; and (e) behaviors in need of activation that would directly oppose avoidance (i.e., opposite-action behaviors). The client is helped to recognize that regular use of this form will not only promote continued progress forward, but will also maintain intervention gains and keep avoidant behavior from reemerging once the formal MAC program ends.

PLAN FOR FUTURE PRACTICE: SELF-REFLECTION AND SELF-CORRECTION

In this final segment of Module 7, the consultant guides the client through a complete review of the Post-MAC Practice Plan form. This form should be systematically completed in the course of Module 7. When reviewing the entire form, the consultant and client should again discuss where the client was and what the client wanted from the MAC program when they began. The efforts that were made, the struggle in which the client inevitable engaged, and the changes made along the way should be pointed out to the client in a fully descriptive way. If the consultant uses the metaphor that the completion of MAC is analogous to graduation, then this last segment of the MAC would be similar to a commencement ceremony. Successes are highlighted, opportunities are identified, and obstacles and personal responsibility for its ongoing success should be noted.

We have consistently taken the position that optimal performance and optimal personal well-being go hand in hand. As such, it is important for the consultant to take this opportunity to note that the skills and practices contained in the MAC have pertained to both personal as well as performance well-being. Continued use and practice of MAC skills as a lifelong process will have benefits well beyond the performance desires with which the client began this program.

Prior to the completion of the MAC protocol, we also suggest that the consultant discuss the unbreakable link between self-reflection and self-correction. One of the underlying principles of the MAC program is that self-awareness leads to self-reflection. This, in turn, leads to the option of choosing self-corrective actions, with all the personal and performance benefits that come with this evolved approach to life. The following vignette clearly illustrates this final segment of Module 7. It may be helpful to refer to the Post-MAC Practice Plan form as you read through the vignette. The client is a 21-year-old collegiate hockey player.

CONSULTANT: So, now that we've gone through each of the parts of the Post-MAC Practice Plan form, let's see how it looks as a whole. Okay, we start with the basic value of being known as a hardworking and reliable player, or, as you put it, a "character guy."

CLIENT: Yeah, this is really what it's all about for me. If I focus on being that kind of person, it seems like the rest would just fall into place.

CONSULTANT: That's great. I think it's important for you to realize just how far you've come in this regard. When we first met, all you wanted to talk about was your next game, and how everyone else was getting in the way of you showing the world how good you could be. (Laughing)

CLIENT: (Laughing) I guess I was a little self-centered. Maybe the best thing I've gotten from all this was a better understanding of what I can control, which is only the choices I make, right?

CONSULTANT: When I take a close look at your Post-MAC Practice Plan form, I notice that you plan on continuing the Brief Centering Exercise and the Mindfulness of the Breath Exercise, both during regular nongame times, between shifts, and between periods.

CLIENT: Yeah, it's really helped. I think I've become really good at noticing stuff going on inside my head really quickly and refocusing when I need to. I think I also feel just more settled. It's hard to put it into words a little, but using these two exercises has made me feel more "peaceful" inside, if that makes any sense.

CONSULTANT: Well, that's a long way from when you told me that the exercises seemed "hokey."

CLIENT: (Laughing) I guess so.

CONSULTANT: I also notice that we put a question mark next to the Task-Focused Attention Exercises. We said we would get back to this later, so I guess now is the time. When we first discussed your future plans for using these exercises, you said that you wanted to use them, but weren't sure how and when.

CLIENT: Yeah, I remember that, and I still think that way a little. These exercises have helped me pay attention when the coach is talking. I used to drift away, especially if I was tired or pissed off, but now, when I notice that I am feeling that way, I can put my attention where it belongs.

CONSULTANT: That's great! Exactly why we include this exercise. But then, why don't you want to continue?

CLIENT: I *do* want to continue to use them, but I am not sure how right now. Honestly, there are no clear situations where my emotions get in the way of my concentration at this point, but I do know that if I begin to notice these types of issues I can practice my focus when I need to. I actually think using the mindfulness exercises helps me in this way on their own.

CONSULTANT: I would expect the mindfulness exercises to work that way, too. That's why the Task-Focused Attention Exercises come later in the program than mindfulness. But, most importantly, you seem to be really aware of yourself. And, you know, that really is the point here. You'll continue to improve as a player and grow as a person if you can stay committed to your values and regularly reflect on your choices. This will keep you flexible and, from that, always able to adjust as your life situation dictates.

CLIENT: Yeah, and actually I *am* concerned about us not meeting anymore. I know we've talked about being able to do this on my own, but you never know.

CONSULTANT: Well, that makes sense for you to wonder about. We did this work together, you have improved in so many ways, and so it is reasonable that you'd ask yourself that question. But, as we know, a thought is not a statement of fact, right? And because you think it, as reasonable as the thought is, it doesn't have to be correct. You can do this on your own. I have no doubt. However, you know I'm still around and you know how to get a hold of me. If an issue arises that is particularly challenging, and you want to bounce stuff off me, just call. But in the meantime, keep working the program.

CLIENT: I knew you'd say something encouraging. (Laughs) You're right, though, and I really do appreciate it.

CONSULTANT: You're welcome. One more comment; I also want to comment that you've clearly identified frustration and anger as emotions that could potentially be an obstacle to doing what you know needs to be done to be the player you want to be. And you indicated that making excuses would be the avoidant behavior. Could you be more specific? What behaviors would the excuses be associated with?

CLIENT: Oh, good question. Let me think about it for a second. (Pause) Okay, well, in the past, when I became frustrated, I would stop listening when the coach was talking, or maybe come late to practice, blow off watching game films, and things like that.

CONSULTANT: Good. I think it is important that you can recognize these behaviors even if you haven't recognized the emotions that are there. Sometimes we can mislabel emotions. We can deny being angry when we are, and just call it stress, which sounds much more noble. So sometimes, the best way to identify what is really going on is to notice the specific behavior that can be a problem.

CLIENT: That makes a lot of sense. I'll fix that on the form. You're right, though, I need to watch for that. And it's funny you said that too, because I used to always say I was stressed when I was really pissed.

CONSULTANT: Well, I think you are ready now. You have come a very long way.

CLIENT: Thanks for the help. I've said before that I'm having the best season I ever had. And my eye's on being named captain next year. That wasn't even close to a possibility a few months ago. I really appreciate everything, it's been an awesome experience.

This vignette demonstrates the review of the Post-MAC Practice Plan form, a review of the key elements of where the player came from and where he thought he was going, some discussion of professional relationship issues regarding the completion of the MAC, and a general sense of the style and form of the discussion. Of particular importance is the clear connection between mindfulness practice and success, as we have regularly noticed that there is a direct relationship between this understanding and success using the MAC protocol.

COMMON PROBLEMS SEEN IN MODULE 7

Only two predictable problems occasionally occur during Module 7. The first relates to observing in the course of Module 7 that the client is not yet ready to complete the program, and thus more sessions are required. This is particularly problematic in a structured environment in which the MAC is being offered in a group format with a predetermined number of sessions. Our strong recommendation in such cases is for the consultant to complete the program as planned and arrange for one additional session at the end of the program with each group or team member to individually discuss his or her gains and remaining needs (just as you would do with an individual client). This affords the consultant the opportunity to discuss post-MAC plans in a private manner and make recommendations regarding any additional intervention needs that may exist. It is not uncommon in group/team settings for it to become clear that some performers in the group/team are experiencing Pdy-related issues that cannot be adequately addressed within the group/team sessions. As such, recommendations made during this final individual meeting may be as simple as constructing post-MAC practice plans or as complex as suggesting the need for additional intervention. We must stress that it is the ethical responsibility to have this discussion and make the necessary suggestions, despite any discomfort that the consultant may feel in these circumstances (Moore, 2003a). When the MAC has been delivered in an individual format, presenting the need for additional sessions is less complex. However, it still requires careful thought and a clear presentation of the reasons for the suggestions, the anticipated number of additional sessions, and the anticipated benefits of continued work. Essentially, the consultant is providing an informed consent for additional sessions. In situations in which the MAC program is presented as an open-ended intervention with no length of time clearly established, this issue becomes obviously less problematic.

The second common problem involves the interpersonal issues that surround program completion and the impact that this has on some clients. This issue is most common with clients experiencing performance dysfunction.

MODULE 7 CONSIDERATIONS FOR WORKING WITH CLIENTS EXPERIENCING PERFORMANCE DYSFUNCTION

During Module 7, there are two related issues the consultant may face when working with individuals experiencing performance dysfunction. The first issue relates to situations in which the basic MAC skills presented during the course of an individually tailored protocol have not been integrated enough to warrant timely termination. As suggested throughout the MAC protocol, it is imperative that the consultant view the seven modules as seven specific learning objectives, which may or may not be most appropriately presented as seven discreet sessions. In the case of individuals who are solely in need of performance development or in cases where the MAC program is being presented to an entire team in a defined period of time, the seven-session format may be most appropriate and/or necessary. However, when the consultant is working with an individual athlete with Pdy, or is working with an entire team in which a specific athlete is experiencing Pdy, a seven-session format may not be appropriate, and decisions regarding the necessary length of treatment must be made on an individual basis.

During Module 7, it is expected that all MAC skills have been practiced and integrated. Yet it is often during this last module when the consultant notices gaps in knowledge or skill that require additional work and thus additional sessions. Gaps in knowledge and skill typically will be noticed during the development of the Post-MAC Practice Plan. In these cases, the performer will not offer many suggestions for future practice and will not be able to easily articulate what skills are in need of particular attention. This is either because the skills have not been adequately developed or because they are not particularly important to the performer's optimal functioning. We therefore strongly encourage the consultant to remain flexible when determining intervention length. In this regard, it may be helpful at the beginning of the protocol to give all clients with performance dysfunction a *range* of the expected number of MAC sessions instead of presenting an absolute number of sessions. Even as late as Module 7, when gaps in knowledge and/or skill are noticed, the consultant should patiently review the specific material and develop a new time frame for intervention completion based on an assessment of the length of time that should rationally be required for additional training in that particular area.

We also suggest that, when MAC skill deficits are noted during the MAC program, it is important for the consultant to evaluate the issues that are blocking skill acquisition. Some questions to ask include: Is it due to lack of practice, perhaps based on avoidance of negative affect or other personal discomfort? Is avoidance present that is based on perfectionism or concerns about displeasing the consultant? Has the performer not fully committed to the program and/or his or her personal development? Are there external factors such as relationship issues that are making it difficult for the performer to invest full effort into the demands of the MAC program? Due to the basic nature of their problem, these and many other issues are particularly likely to be seen among clients experiencing performance dysfunction. In our experience, when MAC skill acquisition has not occurred by this point in the program, it is most often because the client with Pdy does not understand the fundamental connection between the concepts of personal/performance values, experiential avoidance/acceptance, and behavioral commitment. As such, the consultant should evaluate the client's clarity regarding these interrelated concepts before considering any other explanation for the lack of expected MAC skill acquisition.

The second issue often seen among clients with Pdy is related to the completion of the formal component of the MAC program for those who have early maladaptive schemas relating to abandonment and loss. Of course, this schematic issue should have been identified early in the assessment phase of the program, particularly if the consultant used the Young Schema Questionnaire (Young, 1999, 2002) as suggested in chapter 3. If the consultant recognized this issue early in the MAC program, it would be expected that efforts at reinforcing independence and personal responsibility for the success or failure of the MAC program would have occurred. However, even with the consultant's best efforts, this type of schema (as with all schemas) is highly resistant to change, and, as such, nearing the end of formal face-to-face sessions may trigger this early maladaptive schema. The triggering of this schema may not always be obvious. In fact, it can be seen through subtle and/or indirect behaviors such as missing appointments; vague and inconsistent complaints about progress, performance, or relationships; or the instigation of disputes with the consultant over seemingly innocuous events or conversations. When this schema has been previously identified, and when behavior related to this schema is noted toward the end of the MAC program, the consultant should gently but directly confront the behavior as representative of these learned rule systems. While validating this schema by expressing the idea that it is understandable that the client might interpret the world the way he or she does given the client's early life history, the consultant must nevertheless point out the self-defeating nature of the behavior that evolves from this interpretive system and help the client see that, while his or her mind is telling the client something (e.g., the schema-driven thought content relating to loss and/or abandonment), these thoughts do not actually have to reflect reality. Again, thoughts are just thoughts that have been learned to occur in various situations and often do not reflect the reality that the client is confronting. The consultant is thus revisiting the concept of cognitive defusion by helping the client distinguish between thoughts and facts.

The following vignette is an example of a preexisting early maladaptive schema relating to loss and abandonment emerging in the last session of the MAC protocol:

CONSULTANT: Well, we should spend some time preparing your Post-MAC Practice Plan, as we are coming down to the wire of our work together.

CLIENT: I guess. Then you can move on to working with someone else.

CONSULTANT: Well, I work with other people now, and I will continue to in the future. But I am a little confused about why you would say this.

CLIENT: Whatever. It doesn't matter anyway.

CONSULTANT: Actually, it really does.

CLIENT: Okay, well, I was thinking about it during the week, and it seems like as we get closer to the end, all you keep talking about is being finished. So, I guess you're looking forward to it. But that's okay, it's just a job, right?

CONSULTANT: I feel really sorry that you would think that. It *is* my job, but you are suggesting, I think, that I am somehow, and for some reason, looking forward to our work being over. Is that right?

CLIENT: Yes. I guess.

CONSULTANT: Well, given what we learned about your background way back when we began working together, you know, your dad leaving you and your mom when you were an infant, and your mom never demonstrating to you that she cared, I guess you interpreting things this way makes sense, right? And, do you remember when I gave you feedback about those questionnaires you took, and told you about this strong belief that you seemed to have that being abandoned was inevitable for you? I think we are seeing that coming out here.

CLIENT: I remember, but it just seems that way to me.

CONSULTANT: I know it does, but let's consider it for a moment. You have learned this way of thinking about the world, so now, as we get closer to ending the formal part of our work together, suddenly your mind is telling you things that are based on the similarities between your past and what is happening here now. Of course, the differences matter too, and there are major differences. Our professional relationship is very different from the relationships you've had with your family. But what is really most important here is that you remember something we worked on a while back. Remember, when we talked about decentering from your thoughts?

CLIENT: Yeah. That's when we try to see our thoughts as just thoughts.

CONSULTANT: Exactly! The thoughts you are having about my intentions are just thoughts, not realities. And allowing these thoughts to come and go, without acting on them as you began to do at the beginning of today's session can help you focus on what's really going on around you better, because sometimes your thoughts will be correct and sometimes incorrect. The only way to know is to stay connected to the world around you, do what you need to do, and allow time and life to give you all the information you really need.

CLIENT: So you're not trying to get rid of me? (Laughs) I want to know, though, if you kind of care about me as a person?

CONSULTANT: Well, before I answer that I have three questions for *you*. First, what has my behavior throughout the time we have worked together said about that?

CLIENT: It really has seemed that you took a serious interest. You definitely acted like it mattered to you how I was doing.

CONSULTANT: I'm glad to hear that you noticed that. The second question is why would you expect that this would change as we near the end of our work together?

CLIENT: I don't know.

CONSULTANT: Think about it a moment. Your reaction is not based on what I have or haven't done, but on something about the present triggering thoughts about the past. Now, this will always happen to you, and it happens to everyone. It really does happen in different ways for all of us. It is absolutely part of being human, but we can learn to get some distance from what our mind tells us, what we have called decentering, and learn to see our thoughts as just that, stuff that our mind tells us. It doesn't have to mean that what we are thinking is really happening.

CLIENT: I do understand that, but it's really hard to remember all the time. It makes sense, though, and I guess that's why you've been all over me about the idea of mindfulness, because I'm better at seeing that when I am meditating.

CONSULTANT: That's right. Mindfulness practice makes it easier and easier to do this well. But I have one more question. Should whether or not I really care about you affect how you act? Can you still do what's in your best interest regardless of how I think and feel?

CLIENT: (Laughing) Okay, I see where you're going. You're right. I have things to do here for me, and what I want my professional life to be about. I do care how you feel, though, but my actions should be about me and not about your feelings.

CONSULTANT: You got it.

CLIENT: That's what I have to remember. I get upset, though, sometimes, and then it becomes a challenge for me.

CONSULTANT: That does make sense. Just keep this in mind. Okay. Let's go back to our Post-MAC Practice Plan, because that's what we have to make sure you continue to work on.

This vignette demonstrates the impact that specific early maladaptive schemas can have on the termination process within the MAC protocol, and it suggests a strategy for the gentle confrontation of schema-driven behavior along with the integration of previously learned skills and concepts into this important discussion. It should be noted that the consultant in this vignette never actually answered the question about whether he or she cared about the client, because the answer would have provided short-term relief and not the more fundamental change that the MAC program attempts to facilitate. Although this client was relatively easy to work with in this regard, clients with these types of early maladaptive schemas are sometimes very resistant to change and are most likely to require more than one session and more than one conversation to get past the impact of their particular schema.

MAC PROGRAM CONCLUSION

At this point, we are excited to say that the MAC program has been presented in its entirety! Following the theoretical and empirical foundations on which the MAC approach was based, we presented the seven-module

MAC protocol, which can be administered in either individual or group/ team formats. The seven modules are: (1) psychoeducation; (2) introducing mindfulness and cognitive defusion; (3) introducing values and values-driven behavior; (4) introducing acceptance; (5) enhancing commitment; (6) skill consolidation and poise; and (7) maintaining and enhancing mindfulness, acceptance, and commitment. We hope that learning this new intervention approach to performance excellence has been an inspiring journey, and we also sincerely hope that it will change the performance lives of your clients, enhance their overall well-being, and make living each day a more functional, effective, and rewarding experience.

The final three chapters present a detailed case study intended to highlight clients' journeys through the MAC program. The case study in chapter 11 highlights a 21-year-old, Division I female basketball player experiencing performance dysfunction, and chapter 12 highlights a 37-year-old male business executive receiving MAC services for performance development. Both case studies take a comprehensive approach that begins with initial interview and assessment and follows the entire MAC path through all seven modules. Relevant forms, described previously throughout the book, have been completed to demonstrate actual client progress and obstacles. Finally, the case study in chapter 13 describes considerations in the group application of the MAC program. Using 10 members of a men's professional lacrosse team, the chapter highlights the common issues and challenges that accompany group application. Together, these three case study chapters bring the MAC program to life.

PART III

Case Studies

CHAPTER 11

Case Study 1: Performance Dysfunction—The Case of Kayla

Kayla was a 21-year-old African American female basketball player entering her senior year at a major Division I–level university. She had been extensively recruited from a high school in a different region of the United States, following a high school career as a guard in which she was a two-time consensus first-team all-American basketball player. Kayla was a starter and led her team in scoring during all three of her prior collegiate seasons. In addition, her team reached the "Sweet 16" (final 16) in the NCAA tournament in all three of her collegiate seasons. Kayla was also an accomplished student and had chosen to pursue pre-med undergraduate studies.

PRESENTING COMPLAINTS

Kayla was self-referred to the sport psychologist who provided service to the university's athletic department. She requested an individual appointment six games into the basketball season. She described regret about not working out harder during the off-season, which she blamed for a poor start to her current season. In addition, she also reported feeling a great deal of worry over the possibility that she may have a poor season and ruin her chance to be drafted in the first round of the WNBA entry draft. These concerns were leading to many repetitive thoughts about the possibility that she could have compromised the type of professional basketball career that she has dreamed of having. She described spending a great deal of time thinking about these possibilities and stated that she had lost motivation to work hard in both academic and sport domains even though she recognized the self-defeating nature of her choices. Kayla described the first several weeks of the season as "terrible," as both she and her team opened the season poorly. Kayla also indicated that she had recently begun to deal with her worries and concerns by drinking alcohol and partying with friends more than she ever had in the past, which resulted in both poorer conditioning and more concerns about her upcoming season. These behaviors were also creating conflicts with her coach and teammates.

HISTORY AND BEHAVIORAL OBSERVATIONS

Kayla was born in the southeast region of the United States. She comes from an intact family who, she indicates, have been highly involved in her sporting life for as long as she can remember. Kayla described her youth as being essentially happy, but also noted that her mother has always been a "severe worrier," and her father was very strict in his disciplinary style. In addition, she told the psychologist that her father had high expectations for her, even as a small child, and would become angry and distant when she "disappointed him" by not doing as well as she was capable of doing. She is the oldest of three siblings, and her two younger sisters are currently in high school where they both play basketball and hope to receive college scholarships. Kayla reported having a close relationship with both sisters, and reported that they look up to and even idolize her, believing that she represents what they hope to be. Kayla described playing basketball since she was a young child and was told for as long as she could remember that she had the skills and ability to be a professional athlete. In high school, she also ran track, which she described as being primarily for conditioning. However, Kayla acknowledged that she was the best female sprinter on the track team. When asked about her previous basketball performance levels, Kayla acknowledged having brief slumps before, but remarked that they never seemed so bad or resulted in such distress. She described feeling as though her teammates, coach, and father were already disappointed in her and believed that the success or failure of the team was entirely in her hands. Kayla indicated that her parents rarely came to see her play but always insisted on a report via telephone the morning after a game. Kayla noted that, for the first time, she has wondered if she is good enough to play at the professional level and has questioned whether it is worth pursuing. She has thought that she may be better off giving up basketball, working harder to get better grades in school, and making her desired future medical career her top priority. Interestingly, Kayla indicated that she has attained an overall grade point average of 3.75, and was not able to describe how she would or could do better academically if she gave up basketball.

Kayla presented as an attractive, well-groomed, and tall (6'3") woman, who walked and spoke with confidence. She was highly articulate and displayed appropriate affect as she discussed the various topics covered in the interview. Her mood was somewhat dysphoric, which was consistent with her description of feeling sad, and she frequently became teary-eyed during the consultation. When discussing her worries, she became visibly anxious, spoke more quickly, and displayed an overt "leg bounce." When asked for her thoughts about the reason for her poor performance and emotional/behavioral reactions, she blamed a lack of training and commitment. There was little explanation or understanding beyond that.

With Kayla's written permission and following the signing of an appropriate informed consent, the consultant spoke with Kayla's coach. She seemed at a bit of loss to explain Kayla's performance difficulties, but described them as severe enough to consider removing her from the starting lineup. In addition, the coach noted that she had never seen Kayla be so distant with teammates and defiant in response to coaching feedback.

ASSESSMENT

As discussed in chapter 3, preintervention psychological functioning is assessed with a standard clinical interview and a variety of self-report measures. These measures should be selected based on specific processes that appear relevant to the performer's referral question/issue. Based on her presenting concerns, the measures utilized with Kayla included both the athlete and coach versions of the Sport Performance Questionnaire (SPQ; Gardner & Moore, 2006; Wolanin, 2005), the Young Schema Questionnaire-Short Form (YSQ-SF; Young, 1999, 2002), the Penn State Worry Questionnaire (PSWQ; Meyer, Miller, Metzger, & Borkovec, 1990), the Sport Anxiety Scale (SAS; Smith, Smoll, & Shutz, 1990), the Acceptance and Action Questionnaire-Revised (AAQ-R; Hayes, Strosahl, Wilson, Bissett, et al., 2004), and the Beck Depression Inventory-II (BDI-II; Beck, Steer, & Brown, 1996).

The SPQ is a self-report measure that requires the athlete to rate him- or herself on a variety of sport-related behaviors on a 10-point Likert scale. There is a coach version as well, which similarly asks the coach to rate the athlete on the same sport-related behaviors. This instrument was given to Kayla both before and after the MAC intervention and functioned as a measure of intervention outcome with respect to several athletic-related constructs (overall performance, aggressiveness, and concentration). In addition, a variety of measures were utilized to help the consultant gain a more complete and comprehensive understanding of the specific psychological processes that may be impacting Kayla's level of behavioral functioning. In this regard,

- The YSQ-SF was given to evaluate the presence of performance and nonperformance early maladaptive schemas.
- The PSWQ was administered to assess levels of worry.
- The SAS was given to measure sport-related anxiety and concentration.
- The AAQ-R was administered to evaluate the use of experiential avoidance as a characteristic means of responding to (i.e., coping with) unpleasant thoughts and emotions.
- The BDI-II was used to evaluate the current level of depression.

The results of these self-report measures will be discussed within the context of the case formulation presented below.

INITIAL CASE FORMULATION

The case formulation model described earlier was used to organize the case material and assist the consultant in defining the problem to ensure that the MAC program would be the most optimal intervention for Kayla. According to the case formulation model, there are 10 elements that are necessary to consider prior to making an intervention decision: (1) contextual performance demands; (2) skill level; (3) situational demands; (4) transitional and developmental issues; (5) psychological characteristics/performance and nonperformance schemas; (6) attentional focus; (7) cognitive responses; (8) affective responses; (9) behavioral responses; and (10) readiness for change and level of reactance. Each of these 10 specific elements will be discussed in detail as they apply to Kayla.

Contextual Performance Demands

Contextual performance demands refer to the level of competitive demands placed on the performer. Clearly, Kayla was in a highly competitive athletic environment, which had not changed in any significant way during her senior year. There was no reason to believe that contextual performance demands were in any direct way resulting in her performance difficulties.

Skill Level

Skill level refers to the match between performance demands and skill level of the performer. Here again, there was no reason to view Kayla's difficulties as a function of skill deficits. Her basic and advanced basketball skills were judged to be strong by her coach and were good enough for Kayla to be judged to be one of the best female basketball players in the country at the end of her junior season.

Situational Demands

Situation demands refer to the specific situational context in which Kayla is expected to perform her skills. In this case and based on Kayla's own account, it was certainly reasonable to hypothesize that her senior year was the final opportunity to show her skills to scouts and professional organizations before the WNBA entry draft. This resulted in a significant amount of self-induced pressure to perform at optimal levels, making every game, half, and shot more important to her. This pressure increased with each subsequent poor performance.

Transitional and Developmental Issues

Transitional and developmental issues are the natural developmental issues and milestones that are experienced by all humans. In Kayla's case, this would refer to the upcoming conclusion of the college experience (with its normal and expected fears and concerns), exacerbated by the specific fears and concerns related to the difficult goal of pursuing a career in professional sports and the natural pressures and uncertainties that accompany that path. Kayla did not have a personal history of performance adversity until this particular point in time. Her relative lack of experience with adversity accentuated the normal fears and concerns inherent in the pursuit of a career in professional sports, which exacerbated the normal college senior's concerns about life after the relative protection of college and family.

Psychological Characteristics: Performance and Nonperformance Schemas

These psychological schemas refer to the cognitive structures (or verbal rules) that function as a lens by which individuals interpret the world and organize life experiences. The YSQ-SF in particular provided valuable information to help the consultant assess the possible presence of early maladaptive schemas, which may have been contributing to Kayla's emotional and behavioral difficulties. In fact, the YSQ-SF indicated that Kayla manifested very high scores in the early maladaptive schema domain of Impaired Autonomy and Performance, which appeared to be directly related to her presenting complaints. The Impaired Autonomy and Performance early maladaptive schema domain is characterized by an expectation that one will not be able to survive, function independently, or perform successfully in the social or occupational world. Individuals who adopt this internal rule system tend to experience fears and beliefs that center on imminent catastrophe, which may occur and cannot be prevented. This also includes the belief that one is truly incompetent in relation to peers, and it is only a matter of time before everyone will find out.

Attentional Focus

Attentional focus primarily refers to one's direction of attention (self-focused versus task-focused) during performance-related activities. Kayla's description of her most recent performances suggests that she has become increasingly focused on the thoughts and emotions that she experiences while playing, rather than focusing on the basketball-related stimuli and contingencies that are occurring in each and every moment of competition. This appears to be the consequence of early maladaptive schemas being triggered by current situational demands, and has further resulted in overall athletic performance being disrupted. Evidence of attentional difficulties was noted in very low self and coach ratings of concentration on the SPQ, as well as very low scores on the SAS concentration subscale.

Cognitive Responses

Cognitive responses refer to the specific cognitive content—also referred to as automatic thoughts or self-talk—that is experienced during performance-related activities. Kayla reported responding to any poor performance early in a game (i.e., missed open shot, bad pass, missed defensive assignment, etc.) as a trigger for thoughts such as, "Here we go again," "This just keeps getting worse," or "Why do I even bother?" It is important to note that Kayla not only had these random thoughts, but also believed them to be absolutely true. She thus responded to the thoughts as though they were in some way a reality that needed to be addressed.

Affective Responses

Affective responses refer to one's emotional response to performance-related situations. Kayla was clearly responding with high levels of anxiety before games (and she had an elevated score on the SAS anxiety subscale), frustration during games, and sadness and disappointment after games. Kayla interpreted her emotions as evidence of serious problems and proof that her career was "going up in smoke." Consistent with this self-report, her score on the BDI-II suggested mild levels of depression.

Behavioral Responses

Behavioral responses refer to the manner in which an individual responds to the competitive or work situation. Typical styles include active coping and activation of behaviors necessary for improvement and success or avoidance and the associated effort to reduce, eliminate, or otherwise control difficult or painful internal experiences (thoughts and emotions). Kayla was clearly and almost exclusively utilizing experiential avoidance. This was seen in a number of ways. First, she described her effort to control her thoughts by "just not thinking about" those issues that were bothering her, although she noted the ineffectiveness of these efforts. Second, Kayla described increased alcohol use as a way of relaxing and getting away from basketball and all the thoughts and emotions related to it. Third, she reported (later confirmed by her coach) that she did not want to be around her teammates because "They made me think about how I am playing and then I feel bad." Fourth, she was becoming oppositional and defiant in response to coaching feedback, exemplified by statements such as "All the coach's feedback does is make me feel bad, and I feel bad enough, so if I give her a hard time maybe she'll leave me alone." In addition, Kayla's score on the AAQ-R was strongly indicative of extensive experiential avoidance, thus providing psychometric evidence of its presence. Finally, her scores on the SPQ suggested impaired performance in overall performance, aggressiveness, and concentration.

Readiness for Change and Level of Reactance

Readiness for change and level of reactance refer to the client's willingness to acknowledge the need for change, the willingness to make active efforts toward change, and the degree to which he or she is or may become oppositional or defiant in response to suggestion or critique. Kayla's openness to the suggestion that she talk to the consultant and her willingness to discuss her issues and acknowledge that a problem exists suggested to the consultant a level of readiness for change appropriate for the beginning of the MAC program. In addition, it was apparent from her description of the relationship between Kayla and her coach that she certainly had the potential to be somewhat oppositional—a fact that the consultant had to remain aware of as he introduced and ultimately worked through the MAC program.

Extensive Case Description

These 10 elements can be summarized into a complete and comprehensive case formulation to provide a full case description.

Kayla is a young woman who was functioning athletically, academically, and socially at a very high level up to and into her senior year of college. The enhanced transitional and situational pressures relating to the impending end of her college career and expected entry into professional basketball triggered an early maladaptive schema that consisted of strongly held beliefs about her capacity to function independently and adequately (Impaired Autonomy and Performance Schema). This, in turn, exacerbated negative cognitive content (worry and self-doubt) related to this issue and led to associated increases in anxiety, frustration, and sadness. In addition, her attentional focus became increasingly self-focused at the expense of necessary task-focused performance attention. As a means of attempting to scan for and thus control for mistakes, errors, poor performances, and so on, Kayla's primary approach to responding to this negative spiral was extreme avoidance. This avoidance took the form of ineffective efforts at thought suppression, distancing and isolation from teammates, reduced willingness to hear feedback, and increased use of alcohol as a means of dulling uncomfortable affect. The result of this entire dysfunctional process was substantially reduced performance in all life domains. This led Kayla to seek consultation, for which she appeared ready and to which she appeared willing to commit.

According to the case formulation model, the next step is to determine the appropriate MCS-SP classification that best exemplifies the performer's issues. This classification helps the consultant develop an individualized plan for psychological intervention. Utilizing the data accumulated during the assessment phase of service delivery, Kayla's problems appear to be essentially subclinical in nature. Essentially, while still problematic, they do not clearly meet criteria for a formal *DSM-IV-TR* diagnosis (American Psychiatric Association, 2000). Instead, her issues are largely due to the interaction of transitional, situational, and intrapersonal factors. An MCS-SP classification of performance dysfunction (Pdy) was therefore made (Gardner & Moore, 2004b, 2006).

Intervention Planning and Course of Treatment

The intervention plan for Kayla consisted of the MAC program in its entirety. It was determined that Kayla would receive weekly 1-hour sessions for between 7 and 12 weeks (thereby allowing flexibility to work through the seven MAC modules as progress dictated). Kayla agreed to this intervention plan during a post-assessment feedback session in which the case formulation described earlier was presented in detail. It was explained to Kayla that the intervention would not require elimination of troubling thoughts and feelings, because they are a reflection of her personal history and present circumstance. Instead, it was explained that she would develop the ability to notice the presence of these thoughts and feelings without needing to alter them, while retaining (or acquiring) the ability to stay focused on, and committed to, the task at hand. Kayla noted that the formulation made some sense to her, although it was hard for her to believe that the difficulties were not simply a reflection of her finally showing the world that she was simply not good enough.

SESSION 1: PSYCHOEDUCATION

The outline of Module 1 of the MAC program was previously identified as:

1. Introduction
2. Present the Theoretical Rationale for the MAC Program
3. Connect the Rationale to the Client's Personal Performance Experience
4. Explain Automated Self-Regulation of Elite Performance
5. Define Specific Goals of the MAC Training Program
6. Introduce the Brief Centering Exercise

Because Kayla and the consultant had already met, the session began not with introduction, but rather with a discussion of the rationale and purpose of the MAC training along with a discussion of self-regulation and elite athletic performance. Kayla and the consultant carefully went through the description of both functional and dysfunctional performance, with special attention given to the areas in which Kayla was currently having difficulties. Specifically, the problem areas reflecting self-focused attention as directly related to her reduced performance and avoidance as a means of dealing with intrusive and disturbing thoughts and emotions were noted and discussed in some detail. Kayla was open to this explanation and easily grasped the information presented. However, this is not always the case, and often the consultant needs to summarize the model and highlight only those areas that will be the ultimate target of the MAC program. In Kayla's case, she was interested in and grasped the entire model of human performance, which ultimately made the consultant's job substantially easier. When it was clear that Kayla understood the model, the consultant asked her to complete the Performance Rating Form (see Figure 11.1).

Performance Rating Form

Initials: KC   Date: XXXX   Age: 21   Occupation: Student   Gender: Female

Please list performance barriers that have occurred within the last 2 weeks (such as negative thoughts, negative emotions, interpersonal problems, lack of concentration, etc.).

I can't do this. Everyone will see how bad I really am. What am I going to do with my life? How am I going to face my family? I'm ruining my life. I feel so bad I am frustrated and anxious. I feel very sad every day. My teammates hate me and I need to get away from them. I can't concentrate on the court. All I can think about is how I just screwed up or how I'm going to screw up. My form sucks. I'm out of shape.

0	1	2	3	4	5	6	7	8
None		Mild		Moderate		Strong		Extreme

Please rate each of the following using the 0–8 scale above:

Performance Domain	Satisfaction With Performance	Impact of Performance Barrier
Practice/Training	2	8
Competition/Work	1	8
Relationships With Staff	3	8
Relationships With Coworkers/Teammates	2	8
Other (please describe): Schoolwork	4	8

FIGURE 11.1   Kayla's Performance Rating Form

It was clear from Kayla's Performance Rating Form that she believed the barriers noted were having a substantial impact on her overall performance, which included both athletic and school performance. It was also clear that the barriers she noted were consistent with the case formulation noted earlier.

Following a full discussion of the model of human performance (see chapter 1), the consultant moved on to establish the intervention goals of the MAC program. This is a particularly important step, because this is when the MAC intervention goals of enhancing behaviors in the service of basic values is presented. The difficult aspect of this presentation in Kayla's case was when it was suggested that she did not have to reduce, eliminate, or otherwise control her thoughts and emotions, but rather she would develop the ability to become aware of these internal processes and maintain the capacity to focus attention on relevant tasks even when disconcerting thoughts and emotions were present. For Kayla, this was a difficult concept to grasp (as it is for most performers). This is because we are typically taught from an early age that negative thoughts and emotions are bad and must be eliminated or avoided in order for us to do well. Even some sport psychologists who present the notion that optimal performance will occur only in the presence of some "ideal internal state" reinforce the idea that some thoughts or feelings are "bad" and must be eliminated to function optimally. So, when the consultant presented to Kayla the idea that she can feel bad *and* still perform well if her awareness and attention were enhanced and necessary behaviors were activated, she was understandably quizzical. After all, a perusal of her Performance Rating Form clearly indicated a preponderance of "negative" thoughts and feelings. Only after some discussion in which a number of examples from her life were utilized was she able to entertain the idea that optimal performance could occur even when feeling or thinking less than perfectly. Kayla was able to refer to a time in her freshman year of high school when she had similar, albeit less intense, doubts. Yet despite these doubts and anxiety, she performed well. She also noted that she always became anxious and had many negative thoughts when approaching an important academic test, but, despite these thoughts, she was able to focus on the task at hand and generally perform well. The consultant encouraged as many of these examples as possible to solidify and reinforce this critical important point. From this context, the MAC program was outlined and Kayla and the consultant were ready to begin in earnest.

It was at this point of the session that the purpose behind the Brief Centering Exercise was presented and the BCE was practiced, after which the experience was discussed. This exercise was presented as a core component of the MAC, which hopefully over time Kayla would begin to use as a means of nonjudgmentally noticing her many thoughts and emotions while simultaneously redirecting her attention from self to task. Kayla described her first experience with the Brief Centering Exercise as positive. She was able to follow the directions and noted that it was interesting to just notice her thoughts without making any effort to get rid of them (she particularly liked the idea of watching her thoughts as though they were a parade). Kayla also liked the idea that in moving her attention around during the exercise, she was able to be aware of many things rather than simply feel stuck in her thoughts.

After the Brief Centering Exercise, Kayla was given the Preparing for MAC handout, which she was asked to read before the next session. She was also given the What I Have Learned Form, which she was asked to complete as soon as possible after the current session. Interestingly, she chose to complete this form in the hall just outside the office immediately after she left the room.

SESSION 2: MINDFULNESS AND COGNITIVE DEFUSION

The outline of Module 2 of the MAC program was previously identified as:

1. Brief Centering Exercise
2. Discussion of the What I Have Learned Form
3. Check for and Respond to Questions or Uncertainties Regarding the Previous Session
4. Rationale and Importance of Mindfulness
5. Discussion of Between-Session Exercises: What I Have Learned Form, Brief Centering Exercise, and Washing a Dish Mindfulness Exercise
6. Review Session
7. Brief Centering Exercise

Session 2 began with the Brief Centering Exercise, which Kayla indicated that she had used at least once, often twice, a day. The consultant discussed the correct use and common misuse of this exercise, and it was clear that Kayla was using it as a means of developing the capacity to notice her thoughts and direct attention as needed. She appeared to understand the exercise and did not seem to be using it as a means of relaxing or otherwise avoiding thoughts and feelings.

Following the BCE was a discussion of the What I Have Learned Form, which is provided in Figure 11.2. Kayla's What I Have Learned Form shows that she understood the basic message of the first session.

What I Have Learned About Performance and Myself Form

Initials: KC   Date: XXXX   Age: 21   Occupation: Student   Gender: Female

During each session, and across each week of the MAC training program, you are likely to learn a variety of new things about yourself and human performance. After you leave each week's session, I would like you to complete this form as soon as possible. The purpose of this is to ensure that you are learning and remembering the important concepts from each of our sessions together. This allows me to make sure that you are developing all the necessary performance enhancement skills included in the MAC program.

1. My thoughts and feelings don't have to be changed for me to do better in basketball.

2. Thinking about myself too much instead of concentrating on the game in front of me is the biggest problem I have.

3. I can feel bad and still do good.

4. Most of my troubles have come from avoiding rather than dealing with stuff.

FIGURE 11.2   Kayla's What I Have Learned About Performance and Myself Form

Once this became clear, the session moved on to a discussion of the concepts of mindfulness and cognitive defusion. Kayla was asked to complete the Mindfulness Attention Awareness Scale (MAAS; Brown & Ryan, 2003). Presented in chapter 5, this scale is used as a baseline of mindfulness and as a means of objectively noting any improvements in mindfulness during the course of the MAC program. As discussed in chapter 5, mindfulness was described as a central component of enhanced performance through the promotion of enhanced awareness and attention. This is contrasted to the mindless, seemingly automatic manner in which Kayla's negative thoughts and emotions have directed her behavior. Not surprisingly, Kayla's score on the MAAS suggested difficulties with both awareness and attention. In this same context, cognitive defusion was presented as the ability to decenter from her own thoughts or, put more succinctly, to recognize that a thought is just a thought and not an absolute reflection of reality. Kayla was thus presented with the concept that through the systematic and regular practice of mindfulness exercises during the MAC program, she would develop enhanced attention, enhanced awareness of her internal experiences and her environment, and the capacity to recognize a thought as just a thought and still perform as required. Kayla appeared fascinated by this discussion, as most clients are. These concepts, although unlike much of what they have come to think and believe, are very logical and easily connected to personal experience. For performers like Kayla, connecting these concepts with the concept of "flow" (which many performers have heard of in one form or another) is very helpful. In Kayla's case, since she noted that she had heard of flow but did not really understand what it was, this discussion promoted greater interest and a better subsequent discussion.

Following this discussion, the next between-session assignment was presented, which consisted of continued practice of the Brief Centering Exercise and the completion of the Washing a Dish Exercise to be completed three or four times during the coming week. This exercise, presented in chapter 5, was introduced as a means of further developing mindfulness. The exercise utilizes a repetitive task and the client is instructed to focus on the range of sensory experiences (i.e., touch, smell, warmth, sounds, etc.), while becoming aware of the variety of internal experiences that occur simultaneously (such as thoughts and emotions). This was portrayed as the beginning of a series of such exercises that will become more and more relevant to basketball. The goal was simply to perform the exercise and note the experience. Questions to assess include: How easy or difficult was the exercise? Where did your mind take you? What impact did that have on performing the task? How well were you able to refocus? What feelings did you have before, during, and after the exercise? Kayla was also asked to complete the What Have I Learned Form after Module 2.

SESSION 3: INTRODUCING VALUES AND
VALUES-DRIVEN BEHAVIOR

The outline of Module 3 of the MAC program was previously identified as:

1. Brief Centering Exercise
2. Discussion of the What I Have Learned Form
3. Check for and Respond to Questions or Uncertainties Regarding the Previous Session
4. Discussion and Exploration of Values and Values-Driven Versus Emotion-Driven Behavior
5. Additional Home Mindfulness Exercise: Relevant Mindful Activity
6. Discussion of Between-Session Exercises: What I Have Learned Form, Performance Values Form, Given Up for Emotions Form, and Mindfulness Exercises
7. Introduction to Mindfulness of the Breath Exercise

Module 3 began with the Brief Centering Exercise, which allowed a present-moment focus to the session at hand. Following this exercise, Kayla reported continuing to practice this exercise at least once per day, including just before practices and games. In fact, she had begun to use the exercise between halves and just before reentering a game. She reported feeling more attentive and indicated that she "might" be getting better at noticing and letting go of negative thoughts during practice and competition. This was reinforced with a great deal of praise and encouragement, and the consultant pointed out that it sounded like she was doing more than simply using the exercise. She was already beginning to make an effort to view her thoughts as what her mind was saying rather than as facts. Kayla readily agreed and said that she also found herself doing this when she became distracted by self-focused thoughts while studying.

At this point of the session, Kayla and the consultant reviewed her What I Have Learned Form and noted that she again had a solid understanding of the previous week's session. As such, the session moved to a discussion and exploration of the concept of values and how values could and possibly should direct one's actions and choices. This process began with a discussion of the difference between goals and values. It was here that Kayla had some significant difficulties, because she had always seen achievement goals (i.e., winning a championship, leading the league in scoring, becoming a professional athlete) as the only way to define and motivate her. As such, the cross-country travel metaphor noted in chapter 6 was used, and a considerable amount of time was allocated to discussing the difference between values and goals. It was stressed that, while she certainly could, and likely would, achieve many goals in the context of pursuing her values, the pursuit of values was lifelong, defined her as a person, and was not simply a checklist of achievements. The consultant then asked Kayla to complete the Performance Obituary (see Figure 11.3) described in chapter 6.

Although Kayla's Performance Obituary indicated many clear values (i.e., being a hard worker; giving of herself to team, teammates, and the game of basketball; caring about people; and being seen as a championship person), she still indicated a "value" that could be seen as reflecting a (probably unattainable) goal. That is, "she made her family proud of her all the time." Not only was this a *goal* statement much more than a *value* statement, it is also one over which she has no control, because the thoughts, beliefs, and responses of others are not in anyone's control. We then discussed the fact that living a valued life could and probably would make her family proud, but it became apparent that what she really meant was that her family would become proud via her achievements. Kayla quickly recognized this, and, although she began to cry, recognized that this desire was in fact central to many of her current issues. She then modified the Performance Obituary to include living an honest, compassionate, and hardworking life, worthy of her family name. She agreed to post the form inside her locker and read it daily.

This interchange was followed by a discussion of the difference between actions and choices that are directly in the service of values and those that are in the service of emotions. Although, at first, Kayla responded with numerous (and rapid) "I don't know" type of answers indicative of in-session efforts to avoid the topic, she was then able to engage in the discussion and was open to the idea that her drinking, pulling away from others, and many other choices and actions were in the service of her emotions and not her values. Various behaviors previously (during the assessment session) noted as being problematic were discussed, and Kayla was asked to indicate whether they were emotion-driven or values-driven behavior. This was highly effective, because she noted that few of her problems were coming from behaviors that promoted the values that she previously suggested were of importance to her. At this point, Kayla was handed the Given Up for Emotions Form and was asked to complete it for the next session. She was also given the Performance Values Form, which was intended to allow her to clarify her performance values even further. Kayla commented on the amount of forms and then laughingly suggested that it would probably be in the service of her values to complete them all.

This dialogue was followed with a discussion about her experience with the Washing a Dish Exercise. Kayla noted that, at first, she was

Initials: KC   Date: XXXX   Age: 21   Occupation: Student   Gender: Female

What and how would you like your performance/work career and you as an athlete, attorney, salesperson, coworker, teammate, etc. to be remembered?

Kayla was a hard worker, who gave everything she could to her team and the game of basketball. She was a champion in the way she lived her life. She cared about people, and she made her family proud of her all the time.

FIGURE 11.3   Kayla's Performance Obituary

distracted and found it hard to focus on the sensations that were experienced during the dish washing. She also pointed out that she would get bored and frustrated and acknowledged that once she just stopped because it seemed "stupid" to continue. These reactions were discussed as normal responses to the exercise, and this was connected to the fact that the choice to stop was another example of an action in the service of emotion (i.e., boredom) rather than in the service of values (i.e., being a hard worker, giving everything she could to being a basketball player). After this discussion, we agreed on another between-session mindfulness exercise, which was mindful eating. Kayla agreed to eat mindfully, which meant do nothing else while eating. She was instructed to notice all the associated sensations, including smell, taste, and physical sensations. Kayla was also introduced to the Mindfulness of the Breath Exercise and was asked to practice this exercise in addition to the Brief Centering Exercise during the next week.

SESSION 4: INTRODUCING ACCEPTANCE AS AN ALTERNATIVE TO CONTROL

The outline of Module 4 of the MAC program was previously identified as:

1. In-Session Mindfulness Practice
2. Discuss the What I Have Learned Form, Check for and Respond to Questions or Uncertainties Regarding the Previous Session, and Discuss Reactions to the Relevant Mindful Activity Exercise
3. Review Performance Values Form and Given Up for Emotions Form and Pursue Discussion of Obvious and Subtle Avoidance Strategies
4. Experiential Acceptance as an Alternative to Avoidance and the Connection Between Willingness and Values-Driven Committed Behavior
5. Extending the Relevant Mindful Activity Exercise
6. Brief Centering Exercise

Module 4 began with the Brief Centering Exercise, which, according to Kayla, she had begun to effectively use during natural breaks in competitive basketball games. She would take several breaths, focus on her breathing and abdomen rising and falling, and become aware of her thoughts as floats in a parade, which she would subsequently allow to pass and refocus. This was all done in a very brief period of time. Kayla indicated that this was dramatically improving her concentration, and the awareness of her thoughts as simply thoughts was aiding in rapid recovery from errors and other relevant frustrations.

A review of the What I Have Learned Form suggested again that Kayla was effectively incorporating the information presented and discussed during the previous session. She seemed to understand the material and had no questions regarding the previous session. At this point in the session, we moved to a review of the Performance Values Form (see Figure 11.4).

It became obvious when reading through this completed form that Kayla was beginning to make the connection between her internal experiences (emotions and thoughts) and her poor behavioral choices. It was also clear that she was developing the recognition that to pursue her values she would be required to consistently behave in a very specific way despite how she might feel. The material in this form was discussed, and the knowledge and correct connection between values and necessary behavior was strongly reinforced with praise. It was then time to review the completed Given Up for Emotions Form (see Figure 11.5).

During this review, it became clear that, although Kayla was certainly developing a basic understanding of the MAC concepts and was using the material to reduce the frequency of the problematic events, there were still times when her emotions and thoughts were the driving force for her actions. This form was the basis for a discussion of the numerous times during any given week that thoughts or emotions drove her choices. Kayla indicated that these two were just the tip of the iceberg, and, although she believed that she was making progress, there were still many times during a week when she would not recognize how her thoughts and emotions were guiding her behavior until well after the event was over. The consultant tried to normalize this as a natural part of this stage of the MAC program. After all, it was only the fourth session. At this time, the consultant was able to see firsthand Kayla's schemas with regard to disappointing others. She began to cry, as she apologized for being a "bad" client to work with and asked if the consultant would want to "forget the whole thing." The consultant pointed out that it looked like she was doing the same thing in session that she does with coaches and probably family, which is to respond to some evidence of less-than-perfect performance with a strong negative reaction, look for the person to leave (or possibly jump in and save her), and maybe even begin to think about a way out to avoid experiencing the discomfort. This resulted in a long discussion confirming this pattern of behavior. We proceeded to talk about what her mind was telling her and attempted to identify the precise emotional state that she was experiencing, which Kayla noted as being "panicky sad." Because the session time was running out, the consultant asked Kayla to spend some time

Performance Values Form

Initials: KC   Date: XXXX   Age: 21   Occupation: Student   Gender: Female

The following is a list of performance values that may help direct your actions on a daily basis. After each value is recorded, please identify the barriers to, and the actions that must be taken in pursuit of, those values.

Teammate/coworker: What type of teammate/coworker do you want to be? What does it mean to be a good teammate/coworker? Why is being a solid team member/coworker important to you?
I want to be a teammate that can be counted on. I want to be known as someone who works hard and is there to help others. This is what the game is meant to be.

Barriers and Necessary Actions:
My emotions and my worries about myself. I have to put aside my feelings and do what I know is right. Work hard, support teammates, and make them feel appreciated each day.

Sport/Work/Performance Activity: What do you value about your activity? The challenge? Prestige? Enjoyment? Getting to interact with teammates? Helping people?
I love playing basketball. Everything about it. It feels like the world stops for me when I'm on the court.

Barriers and Necessary Actions:
When I start thinking about how good or bad I'm doing, and worry about my future in pro basketball. I have to focus on the game itself and find the enjoyment in every minute on the court.

Training: Is developing your skill important to you? Why is working at getting better meaningful to you? Are there any skills you'd like to learn or develop more fully?
I take pride in my game and I know that I have to get better at every-thing, every aspect of my play needs some work.

FIGURE 11.4   Kayla's Performance Values Form

Barriers and Necessary Actions:
When I get too worried, I don't feel like playing and then I find something else to do because I don't want to deal with it. I'd rather chill than deal with the frustration and anxiety. I know I have to work hard no matter how I feel. Go to practice, smile, interact, and play.

Technical Skills: What issues or behaviors related to technical skill development do you care about (e.g., time spent working on golf swing, sales presentation skills, etc.)? What would you like to do more of?
I need to spend time working on shooting from 3-point range.

Barriers and Necessary Actions:
Not wanting to deal with how I feel and just not practicing, or practicing the easy stuff. I guess I have to put time aside because it really matters, and stick to it no matter what.

Tactical Skills: What issues or behaviors related to tactical skill development do you care about (e.g., effort spent on planning a sales or presentation strategy, developing greater understanding of pitch or club selection, situational play, etc.)? What would you like to do more of?
Coach says I can use some work in seeing the need for offensive spacing on the court.

Barriers and Necessary Actions:
Not wanting to deal with the criticism that she puts on me about this. I guess I need to approach her directly and find out what she thinks I need to do, film work or whatever.

Recreation/Fun: What type of activities do you enjoy? Why do you enjoy them?
Just hanging out with my friends, watching movies and television.

Barriers and Necessary Actions:
Sometimes I don't give myself permission to relax. It's like if you don't do well, you don't deserve time to chill.

FIGURE 11.4 Continued.

Given Up for Emotions Form

Initials: KC   Date: XXXX   Age: 21   Occupation: Student   Gender: Female

The purpose of this form is to help you become more aware of what you have given up to reduce or eliminate your emotions. What opportunities in the service of your values are you giving up in the service of feeling less emotion? How is this affecting your ability to perform better and enjoy your competitive/work world more?

In the first (far left) column, list a situation related to practice, training, or actual competition/work that triggered a strong emotion. In the second column, write down the specific emotion that was experienced. In the third column, record what you did to reduce or satisfy your emotion. In the fourth column, write down what your effect efforts to control or reduce your emotion had on you. In the last (far right) column, write down the long-term consequences of your efforts to rid yourself of these emotions (what you gave up to reduce or satisfy your emotion).

Complete form below:

Situation or event	Emotion	What you did to control emotion	Short-term effect	Long-term effect on you
Missed first 3 shots in the game	Frustration	At first tried not to think about it	It didn't work and I yelled at a teammate	My shooting gets worse as the game goes on
Coach said at this rate I would never play pro ball	Angry and sad	Began to walk off the court, but then stopped myself	Didn't have to deal with it	Relationship with coach would get worse. Bad reputation

FIGURE 11.5   Kayla's Given Up for Emotions Form

focusing on the feelings that she was experiencing and describe them in detail. The purpose was to begin the process, to be continued next week, to accept the emotional experience, to fully experience it without the need to run away, and from there to develop the willingness to have the emotion and still do what is necessary in any given moment. After several minutes of describing her emotions in detail (i.e., physical sensations, where it was experienced, etc.), the consultant told Kayla that she was doing a good job just sitting with the emotion and that the session would end with a 10-minute Mindfulness of the Breath Exercise to help her have and notice these uncomfortable thoughts and feelings without judging them.

After this exercise, Kayla reported still feeling badly but was somewhat more focused and ready to continue her day. She was asked to complete the Given Up for Emotions Form again, continue to practice her mindfulness exercises, and complete the What I Have Learned Form prior to the next session. Because we were only able to complete the first half of Module 4, session 5 would be focused on completing this module rather than beginning Module 5. This is an example of the flexibility of the modular MAC program—any module can be delivered as either a single session or multiple sessions based on the circumstances and needs of the client.

SESSION 5: INTRODUCING ACCEPTANCE AS AN ALTERNATIVE TO CONTROL (CONTINUED)

After performing the Brief Centering Exercise, session 5 (the second half of Module 4) began just as session four had ended, with a discussion of the effects of emotion. The conversation focused not on the direct effects of the emotion, but rather on the indirect effects. Kayla and the consultant talked about specific behaviors such as leaving the court, talking back to the coach, yelling at teammates, and a number of other similar behaviors that were the real problem. From this point, we talked about the various ways that avoidance, both obvious and subtle, can impact the ability to pursue values. Kayla was soon able to see that emotion was not the problem, but, in fact, the problem was all the things that she did and tried to do to avoid, escape from, eliminate, reduce, or in some way control emotions. At this point, the idea of acceptance was introduced, which is the idea that one can have (i.e., accept) emotions as a natural part of life, with no need to make them go away or lessen them in any way. This was followed by a review of her Given Up for Emotions Form, which again contained two entries, very similar to the previous week. In one entry, her frustration with herself resulted in running back into a defensive position after a missed shot so slowly that she was benched for the remainder of the half. The other entry described her becoming sullen and withdrawn in practice when confronted with an error. When this form was reviewed, the discussion focused on how it would be different if Kayla were willing to have her emotions with no need to avoid or escape them—to accept feeling bad, notice her thoughts and emotions, and refocus on the task at hand *while* feeling badly. We formulated the different behaviors that would follow from this way of viewing the world, and Kayla recognized that this approach would be completely in the service of her values and not intended for short-term comfort. This concept was discussed as equivalent to the word *poise,* and the consultant stressed the importance of developing poise in the context of enhanced performance. Kayla appeared to understand the concept, a little easier than most clients, and seemed eager to get to work on becoming willing to have her emotions become separate from her behavior.

The consultant engaged in a discussion of her mindfulness practice, and how it related to the concept of acceptance. Kayla noted that she had to be aware of her emotions before she could work at accepting and not avoiding and was easily able to recognize the role of mindfulness practice in this endeavor. She also seemed to understand and report tangible benefits of mindfulness as a means of decentering from her thoughts. In this regard, she reported improvements in becoming aware of her thoughts—especially thoughts relating to pleasing others—while not believing that she had to act on them. We then discussed using more performance-related mindfulness activities and developed a hierarchy of times when mindfulness practice, either by way of the Brief Centering Exercise or mindfulness activities (similar in concept to Washing a Dish or mindful eating), would be appropriate. She identified prepractice and pregame stretching, warm-up drills, foul shooting practice, and when sitting on the bench and waiting to come back into the game as good times. Kayla agreed to work another of these relevant mindfulness activities into her routine and expressed a belief that it would not only help her enhance attention, but would also allow her to be more aware of the emotions that often trigger her self-defeating behaviors.

The session ended with Kayla being asked to regularly check out her Performance Values Form to reconnect with what she really wanted basketball to be for her. She was again given the Given Up for Emotion Form to complete before the next session and was asked to complete the Emotion and Performance Interference Form as well. In addition, a brief review of her previous mindfulness assignment was undertaken, and the session ended with the Brief Centering Exercise.

SESSION 6: ENHANCING COMMITMENT

The outline of Module 5 of the MAC program was previously identified as:

1. In-Session Mindfulness Practice
2. Review of Previous Session
3. Enhancing Commitment: Connecting Values, Goals, and Behaviors
4. Review and Assign Performance-Relevant Mindfulness Homework
5. Session Review and Brief Centering Exercise

Moving into Module 5 of the MAC program, the emphasis began to shift toward activating specific behaviors relevant to Kayla's performance values.

Session 6 began with a 15-minute Mindfulness of the Breath Exercise, followed by a brief review of Kayla's continuing use of mindfulness exercises. Her mindfulness practice was regular and frequent, and Kayla reported seeing enhancement in both attention and awareness. Although she indicated that she still had a way to go in this regard, Kayla indicated that the increase in awareness was helpful in noticing yet not acting on a variety of thoughts and emotions, and that the enhanced attention was helpful in remaining focused in competitive situations.

Following the mindfulness exercise and discussion, the session moved on to a review of her between-session Given Up for Emotions Form, on which she listed three mid-competition events where she noticed her emotion (in each case, frustration), noticed her "negative" thoughts, and quickly refocused and extended "extra" effort to "do the right thing." Following this, Kayla and the consultant reviewed her completed Emotion and Performance Interference Form (see Figure 11.6).

The consultant first asked Kayla if only two events such as this really happened, because he had expected to see many more situations. She responded by suggesting that she had her best week in a very long time and that, although neither of these two situations resulted in any performance disruption, they were the only two that even came close. The manner in which Kayla completed the form and discussed her week suggested to the consultant that she was being forthcoming and, as such, she was reinforced for both having a "good week" and (more importantly) clearly working the program.

With the basic skills and concepts of mindfulness, cognitive defusion/decentering, and acceptance/willingness as a replacement for avoidance seemingly in place, the discussion then turned to the connection between

	Emotion and Performance Interference Form		

Initials: KC   Date: XXXX   Age: 21   Occupation: Student   Gender: Female

Please record performance situations that occurred during the past week, the emotion(s) experienced, the degree to which these emotions interfered with performance, and how these emotions interfered with performance.

Situation	Emotion Rate Intensity 0 = none 10 = extreme	Performance Interference Rate Intensity 0 = none 10 = extreme	What Happened?
Coach got on me at practice	Anger/7	Started to sulk/4	Stopped myself and pushed ahead
Great first half, then missed first 2 shots and turned the ball over	Anxiety/5	Became preoccupied/5	Quickly refocused

FIGURE 11.6   Kayla's Emotion and Performance Interference Form

values, goals, and defining specific behaviors needing to be activated on a daily basis. With her values clearly recorded and frequently revisited as an anchor for her actions and choices, Kayla and the consultant identified her goals, which she defined in terms of personal success (lead conference in scoring, all-American selection, first-round draft choice), team success (NCAA Final Four), and interpersonal success (being voted best team player by her teammates). We discussed how these goals may occur within the context of her values and noted that she really did not have to spend much time focusing on these goals if she engaged in values-directed behavior on a day-to-day basis. This naturally led to a discussion of what specific behaviors were necessary and how she could demonstrate commitment (which was defined as *doing* in the service of values rather than just *wanting* things to turn out well) by activating these behaviors. Kayla attempted to define these specific behaviors. The specific behaviors identified were as follows:

a. Getting to practice on time.
b. Working as hard as she could in practice on the areas where she is weakest.
c. Being the last one to leave the court at the end of practice every day.
d. Making a point to help a teammate in some way every day.
e. Regularly completing physical training (including eating right) and MAC-related mental training.
f. Reaching out to her coach to seek advice and assistance.

Kayla was asked to write down these behaviors within the Committing to Performance Values Exercise and record her activation of these behaviors in the appropriate place on the form (see Figure 11.7). We then discussed the importance of becoming increasingly willing to experience negative thoughts and emotions while pursuing her values and striving for her goals.

Following a lengthy discussion of the connection between willingness, behavioral commitment, values, and goals, it was time to move on to the next portion of session 6 (still Module 5), which was the continued discussion of her performance-relevant mindfulness exercises. During the previous week, Kayla engaged in Mindfulness of the Breath while stretching, warming up, and between periods, and she performed the Brief Centering Exercise during her pregame routine, while on the bench just after being taken out and just before going back into the game, and during time-outs. It was suggested that the natural next step would be to use the Brief Centering Exercise (which she could now effectively utilize in as little as 10 seconds) during appropriate natural breaks in

Committing to Performance Values Exercise

Initials: KC   Date: XXXX   Age: 21   Occupation: Student   Gender: Female

Performance Value (PV):
Being known as a hardworking and reliable athlete, who put everything that she could into the game of basketball.

Short-Term Goal Associated With PV:
Improving conditioning and basketball performance (particularly 3-point shooting percentage) leading up to the WNBA draft.

Long-Term Goal Associated With PV:
Regaining respect of coaches and teammates, becoming recognized as a leader.

Behavior To Be Added or Changed To Achieve PV:
Getting to practice on time, working as hard as she can in practice on the areas that she is weakest, and being the last one to leave the court at the end of practice every day.

Situation:

_____

_____

Action Taken:

_____

_____

FIGURE 11.7   Kayla's Committing to Performance Values Exercise

play, particularly following a mistake or poorly executed play of some kind. After a discussion about how this might work and times when it would not be applicable, the session concluded with the Mindfulness of the Breath Exercise.

SESSION 7: SKILL CONSOLIDATION AND POISE: COMBINING MINDFULNESS, ACCEPTANCE, AND COMMITMENT

The outline of Module 6 of the MAC program was previously identified as:

1. In-Session Mindfulness Exercises
2. Review of Previous Session
3. Putting It All Together: Enhancing Poise Through Exposure-Based Activities
4. Review and Assign Performance-Relevant Mindfulness and Task-Focused Attention Exercises
5. Brief Centering Exercise and Review of Between-Session Forms

Session 7 (Module 6 for Kayla) began with the Mindfulness of the Breath Exercise and a discussion of the week's events. Kayla reported having her best basketball week for the season, and was named conference player of the week. She also reported doing much better at school and, most importantly to her, was focusing better at everything she was doing. As she said, "I am more focused when I'm eating, driving, studying, and playing ball." Kayla attributed this to enhanced mindfulness skills along with increasing skill at noticing and letting go of thoughts representing self-focused attention. Although this was out of the typical session sequence for this module of MAC, the consultant continued from this point to a discussion of the previous week's session and a review of the between-session assignments that Kayla had been asked to complete. Kayla showed the consultant the list of behaviors to be activated in the service of her values and goals (determined during the previous session) and noted that each specific behavior was activated multiple times during the week. This was strongly reinforced by the consultant, and Kayla went on to note that she frequently acted in the service of her values even when she was feeling something that would have previously led to avoidant behavior. Kayla was particularly proud of this and strongly believed that this signified a major step in her development.

Following that very positive discussion, the concept of the Task-Focused Attention Exercise was presented. As noted in chapter 9, this exercise was presented to Kayla as one that will help further develop her

capacity to redirect attention away from the self and one's internal processes such as thoughts and emotions and back to the relevant external
task at hand. The exercise was presented as being similar to mindfulness,
in that awareness of the direction of attention is enhanced, and the ability to focus fully on all aspects of a particular situation is optimized. It
was also suggested that the exercise differs from mindfulness in that it is
intended to allow for purposeful attentional redirection *during* difficult
situations, whereas mindfulness is intended to simply notice internal processes and allow attention to essentially move itself.

After ensuring that Kayla understood the purpose of the exercise,
she and the consultant completed it as described in chapter 9. After the
first run-through of the exercise, Kayla remembered about 25% of
the material presented. Kayla was surprised at how poorly she did and
indicated that it was hard for her to focus on the consultant's voice while
worrying about how well she would do. We discussed the similarity of
this reaction to many performance situations that she faces, and Kayla
added that recently she "zoned out" during a time-out, thinking about
"who knows what" while her coach was giving instructions. Later,
when she was on the court, she made a mistake because she did not hear
what she was really supposed to do. Given this discussion, Kayla both
understood the point of the exercise and recognized its value. Two more
run-throughs were then completed and she systematically increased her
percentage remembered to near 90%. Interestingly, and importantly,
Kayla noted that, each time she did the exercise, she became more and
more nervous, because she was concerned about her performance. However, she was able to allow that emotion to exist and still focus her attention externally on the information that was being conveyed to her. The
discussion then focused on ways in which she could practice this between
sessions. Kayla came up with sitting in a noisy room, spending 20 seconds looking around, and then closing her eyes and writing down everything she could remember seeing in the room. She saw this extension of
the exercise as related to basketball (seeing the entire court) and at the
same time as enhancing external focus of attention.

Following this, we discussed the importance of confronting the most
difficult or emotionally charged situations and learning to remain in those
situations until the emotion abated or until one is able to function the
way one needs to (exposure). After a brief discussion of the concept and
the value, Kayla made a short list of emotionally evocative situations that
she still avoided. The two major items on the list were: (1) talking and
apologizing to her coach and her teammates about her previous behavior and (2) talking to her father about the way his attitude in response
to poor performance results in a distance between the two of them. We
talked about the need to remain in the situation for as long as possible to

make sure that everything that needs to be said is said regardless of her emotional state during the conversations, and calmly remaining in the situation *even* if the people that she interacts with respond badly in any way. Kayla and the consultant discussed how this type of activity (which would be a form of exposure) is directly related to poise, which was again defined as the ability to function in the way that one wants and needs to function *despite* one's immediate thoughts and emotions. We discussed what her mind might tell her in each situation, what emotions were likely to be experienced, and, most importantly, how these actions were directly in the service of her stated values.

Kayla's performance-relevant mindfulness assignments were reviewed, which she described as going very well. Kayla reported using these exercises in each of the situations that she listed during the previous session, except for during natural breaks in play. She established this as her assignment for the following week. Given her progress, we discussed that we had to decide how many additional times we needed to meet in the formal part of the MAC program. The consultant pointed out that there was one session left on the formal agenda, although additional sessions could be made available if deemed necessary. The consultant also pointed out that Kayla had achieved most of what was set out to be accomplished, and that after the formal program was over, the consultant would be available through the athletic department if any additional issues arose. Kayla became quiet for a few moments, and then said that, while she would miss attending the sessions, she thought that one additional session was probably enough for her. Of course, this would be based on whether the objectives of the seventh MAC module were completed in one session.

After the Brief Centering Exercise to conclude the session, an appointment was scheduled for 2 weeks rather than the usual 1-week interval to gauge Kayla's use of her MAC skills at a slightly longer interval.

SESSION 8: MAINTAINING AND ENHANCING MINDFULNESS-ACCEPTANCE-COMMITMENT

The outline of Module 7 of the MAC program was previously identified as:

1. Review Previous Session and Overall MAC Program
2. Brief Centering Exercise
3. Task-Focused Attention Exercise
4. Review of Current Level of Experiential Acceptance, Willingness, and Commitment to Values
5. Plan for Future Practice: Self-Reflection and Self-Correction

Following the Brief Centering Exercise, Kayla and the consultant spent a few minutes reviewing both the previous session and the entire MAC program experience. Kayla suggested that the program was much better than she had hoped for and that she felt as though she "got [her] life back" from the sessions. She indicated that engaging in mindfulness and all that was connected to it was probably the most helpful, although she also indicated that focusing on behaving in a manner consistent with her values had become central to the way she thought about her day-to-day life. Kayla indicated that she had been taking the concept of poise very seriously and that she had spent a good deal of time in conversations with her coach, a number of teammates, and even her father. She reported that these conversations, especially the conversation with her father, were very uncomfortable but that she handled them with a great deal of poise. When asked what she meant, she indicated that to her it meant "feeling bad but still doing it," and doing it well. Kayla suggested that she doubted anyone could really tell just how anxious she was during each conversation. She went on to talk about several on-court events that she handled with poise and indicated that her current level of basketball performance was as good if not better than it has ever been.

The consultant asked Kayla to complete several of the self-report measures used during the preintervention assessment phase. She was asked to complete the BDI-II, the AAQ-II, the SPQ, and the PSWQ. The results of these self-reports indicated a nonclinical level of depression, improvements in the AAQ such that experiential avoidance could no longer be viewed as a problematic process, a reduction in worry to a nonclinical level (PSWQ), and performance ratings on the SPQ suggestive of superior self-ratings of performance. In addition, she was asked to complete the MAAS to assess her enhanced mindfulness skills. Her score suggests that she had significantly enhanced her skills in mindful awareness and mindful attention, as she had reported.

Finally, the Performance Rating Form first administered during session 1 was readministered (see comparative results shown in Figure 11.8).

It is apparent that Kayla made significant improvements in both performance outcomes and the psychological processes (i.e., enhanced attention, enhanced mindfulness, reduced avoidance) that account for enhanced performance and that are at the foundation of the MAC program. The consultant and Kayla reviewed these results, which confirmed her own report. In addition, she handed the consultant a sealed letter from her coach, which we read together. In the letter, the coach indicated that the improvements in performance and, possibly more importantly, in Kayla's approach to people, friends, and school were so marked that it was "like another human being had shown up in her place." Kayla

Performance Rating Form: Session 1

Performance Domain	Satisfaction With Performance	Impact of Performance Barriers
Practice/Training	2	8
Competition/Work	1	8
Relationships With Staff	3	8
Relationships With Coworkers/Teammates	2	8
Other (please describe): School work	4	8

Performance Rating Form: Session 8

Performance Domain	Satisfaction With Performance	Impact of Performance Barriers
Practice/Training	10	2
Competition/Work	10	1
Relationships With Staff	8	3
Relationships With Coworkers/Teammates	9	2
Other (please describe): School work	9	3

FIGURE 11.8   Kayla's Performance Rating Form: Comparative Results From Session 1 and Session 8

became teary-eyed in response, feeling badly for where she had been and the time she had lost and at the same time feeling extremely good about where she had arrived.

At the completion of the MAC program, Kayla no longer met criteria for a performance dysfunction classification. She was no longer complaining about performance difficulties, was no longer experiencing psychological distress, and was responding to her world in more effective and flexible ways—all consistent with the essential goals of MAC.

Completing the session included one more Task-Focused Attention Exercise, which involved both remembering orally presented details and also remembering the physical details of the room. This was effectively completed, with Kayla remembering nearly 100% of the orally presented details and remembering a large number of visual details. Kayla reported practicing this exercise between sessions as she had planned to do during the last session, and she indicated that it was having a significant positive effect on her attention to task.

We concluded the session by reviewing her values, the specific behaviors connected to those values, and the barriers that would be ever-present in her life. From this perspective, a 2-month plan to continue working on these skills was developed. It included continued use of the Committing to Performance Values Exercise that she would use on a regular basis to keep track of the behaviors in the service of her values that she regularly activates. Kayla indicated that she would keep a "MAC training log" and include all of these activities to review and monitor regularly. We discussed the potential availability of the consultant for informal review of this log and/or follow-up sessions if needed. The consultant reminded her of the need to regularly practice and stay focused on decentering from thoughts and remaining committed to her values. Kayla indicated that working on being attentive and poised had become increasingly important to her, which she recognized could only be achieved through ongoing attention to the values that defined her life as a basketball player and a person. Of course, both the session and the overall MAC program ended with the Mindfulness of the Breath Exercise.

CHAPTER 12

Case Study 2: Performance Development—The Case of Daniel

Daniel was a 37-year-old White male and a senior executive at a large publicly held Fortune 500 U.S. company. Daniel received his bachelor of arts degree from a prestigious university on the West Coast of the United States and had been employed by his present company since graduation. He currently held the position of senior vice president for account development and was on the executive council of his company. This council included the chief executive officer (CEO), the chief financial officer, and three senior vice presidents. The council served as the executive team and was responsible for managing both the day-to-day functioning and long-term planning for the company. Daniel was the youngest member of the executive council and had been promoted to his current position in an extremely quick period of time. The chairman of the board of directors had told Daniel that he was viewed as the future CEO of the company. Daniel reported that he had been "ultra successful" in every facet of his business life and was happily married and living with his wife of three years in a large suburban home.

PRESENTING COMPLAINTS

Daniel was referred to the consultant by a friend of his who had previously utilized the consultant's services. He described himself as "feeling stuck," which he described as the belief that he had gone as far as he could

231

go without improving in fundamental areas in his life. Specifically, as he had risen through the corporate ranks, he at times thought that he really wasn't deserving of the promotions and that, sooner or later, upper management would realize this and he would lose everything. In response to these thoughts, Daniel would become "tense" and would begin to avoid his busy workday in some subtle ways. For example, he reported frequently taking extra time for lunch, putting off making uncomfortable phone calls in which he would have to give bad news to people reporting to him, and not responding to e-mails or telephone calls, only to have them pile up. The consequences of these avoidant behaviors led Daniel to feel quite overwhelmed. In turn, this avoidance led to severe self-recrimination and resulted in brooding at home and disconnection from his wife. Although she interpreted Daniel's behavior as a reflection of his personality, it often resulted in her becoming unhappy. Daniel reported that these issues, while intermittent and not particularly severe, were still uncomfortable and led to serious concerns about his capacity to handle any further promotions.

HISTORY AND BEHAVIORAL OBSERVATIONS

Daniel was born in southern California to a working-class family. He described a close relationship with his mother and father, who were both retired, and a younger sister who was married to an advertising executive in the Midwestern United States. Daniel reported doing consistently well in all levels of school and majored in business management in an academically challenging university. Upon graduation, Daniel took an entry-level sales position in his current company and rapidly moved through the corporate ranks with significant salary increases along the way.

Daniel indicated that he has always been very hard on himself and had long believed that he was "not as bright" as his peers in college. He also believed that he performed well only due to extremely hard work. He stated that this old belief sometimes currently affected him. For example, he stated that, when in executive council meetings, he was sometimes reticent to state contrary opinions for fear that, as someone not as "smart" as others in the room, he should perhaps keep his thoughts to himself and not risk appearing "dumb." Daniel indicated that this issue increased as he climbed the corporate ladder, and was thus a more serious issue than it had been in the past. He also realized that he must overcome this issue in order to demonstrate the decision-making and leadership ability necessary for an even higher senior position.

Daniel presented as a tall (6'1"), attractive man who was well dressed at the time of the interview. He demonstrated a full and appropriate range of affect, reported no extreme distress, and appeared to be quite insightful relating to his present reason for seeking consultation.

ASSESSMENT

Preintervention psychological functioning was assessed with a standard semistructured interview and three self-report measures selected based on specific processes that appeared most likely to be relevant to the performer's referral issue. The measures utilized included the Young Schema Questionnaire-Short Form (Young, 1999) to assess for the presence of relevant early maladaptive performance and non–performance-related schemas, the Acceptance and Action Questionnaire-Revised (Hayes et al., 2004) to assess for the presence of experiential avoidance, and the Profile of Mood States (McNair, Lorr, & Dropplemen, 1971) to assess the levels of negative mood experienced by Daniel at the time of interview. The results of this assessment will be presented within the case formulation described below.

INITIAL CASE FORMULATION

The case formulation model (Gardner & Moore, 2006) was used to organize the case material and assist the consultant in defining the presenting problem to ensure that the MAC program would be the appropriate intervention for Daniel.

Again, within the case formulation model, there are 10 components that are necessary to consider before making an intervention decision: (1) contextual performance demands; (2) skill level; (3) situational demands; (4) transitional and/or developmental issues; (5) psychological characteristics/performance and nonperformance schemas; (6) attentional focus; (7) cognitive responses; (8) affective responses; (9) behavioral responses; and (10) readiness for change and level of reactance. Each of these 10 components will be discussed in detail.

Contextual Performance Demands

Contextual performance demands refer to the level of performance demands placed upon the performer. It was apparent that Daniel was in a highly competitive and intense corporate environment. Daniel's promotion several years ago intensified this fact, but the demands placed upon him had not recently changed.

Skill Level

Skill level refers to the match between performance demands and skill level of the performer. There was no reason to view Daniel's presenting issues as a function of skill deficits. Daniel reported that his fundamental and more corporate-specific business skills were judged to be excellent, as evidenced by superior semiannual performance reviews. He presented these reviews to the consultant. In addition, his skills and performance were strong enough for Daniel to be seen as a possible future corporate CEO.

Situational Demands

Situation demands refer to the specific situational context in which Daniel is expected to perform his skills. Certainly, by any measure, Daniel's job situation was relatively stable with no unexpected or time-specific situation that was placing additional demands on his performance.

Transitional and Developmental Issues

Transitional and developmental issues are the natural developmental issues and milestones that are experienced by all humans. In Daniel's case, this would refer to the promotional path that he has had and expects to have in the future. Daniel was in a period of his life when he was both reflecting upon his past and considering the realistic expectations for the future. For Daniel, the consistency with which he has excelled, with the expectation of a continued rise into the upper echelon of corporate life, created a unique stress for this otherwise well-functioning individual.

Psychological Characteristics: Performance and Nonperformance Schemas

These psychological characteristics refer to the cognitive structures (or verbal rules) that function as a lens through which individuals interpret the world and organize life experiences. The YSQ-SF was used to assess the possible presence of early maladaptive schemas, which may have been contributing to Daniel's stated difficulties. Although the YSQ-SF indicated that Daniel had no clinically relevant elevations in any early maladaptive schema domain, he did manifest slightly elevated scores on the early maladaptive schema domains of *overvigilance* and *other-directedness*. These schemas suggested that Daniel had set extraordinarily high standards for himself and that he may have, at times, been excessively concerned with how others viewed him. Both of these slight elevations were consistent with his stated concerns.

Attentional Focus

Attentional focus refers to the direction of the performer's focus of attention (self-focused versus task-focused) during performance-related activities. Daniel's description of himself suggested that he was able to maintain task focus when involved in his work and did not typically become distracted.

Cognitive Responses

Cognitive responses are the specific cognitive content—also referred to as automatic thoughts or self-talk—that are experienced during performance-related activities. Daniel reported wondering when others would recognize that he is not as good as everyone thinks, and would on occasion tell himself that he is really not up to the challenge of being in such a high-level position.

Affective Responses

Affective responses are the emotional responses to performance-related situations. Daniel indicated that he was becoming "tense" more frequently at work and at home. Consistent with this self-report, his score on the POMS suggested minor elevations of *tension,* but suggested that his overall mood was well within normal limits during the most recent 2 weeks.

Behavioral Responses

Behavioral responses refer to the manner in which the individual responds to his or her experiences in performance situations. Typical styles include either active coping and activation of those behaviors necessary for improvement and success or avoidance and the associated effort to reduce, eliminate, or otherwise control difficult internal experiences. Daniel was increasingly utilizing experiential avoidance as a means of responding to the increased pressure that he was experiencing. This avoidance was seen in a number of ways: (1) he described increases in the number of times that he would extend his lunch breaks to avoid stressful tasks; (2) he occasionally avoided calling or meeting with individuals he managed when having to deliver bad news; and (3) he increasingly avoided reading e-mails and checking telephone messages to avoid extra stress. Consistent with these reports, Daniel's score on the AAQ-R revealed a moderate level of experiential avoidance.

Readiness for Change and Level of Reactance

Readiness for change and level of reactance refer to the performer's willingness to acknowledge the need for change, the willingness to make active efforts toward change, and the degree to which the client is or may become oppositional or defiant in response to suggestion or critique. Daniel was self-referred and gave every indication that he was willing to work on developing the skills necessary for enhanced performance. Neither his history nor his presentation style suggested oppositional or defiant behavior in response to suggestion or criticism.

EXTENSIVE CASE DESCRIPTION

Summarizing the 10 elements into a comprehensive case formulation provides the following case description:

Daniel was a high-functioning adult male who has demonstrated consistent levels of performance throughout his life time. Although he currently desired to enhance his work performance and in particular develop the skills required for more advanced future positions within his company, there was no evidence to suggest that Daniel's performance had degraded in any significant way. In addition, there was no evidence to suggest that either external or internal factors were at the core of his desire for enhanced performance. Some very mild levels of early maladaptive schema were present and needed to be bypassed in the pursuit of enhanced performance, but these schemas were neither significant nor overarching in their impact on his career direction or his overall personal well-being. Rather, it appeared that Daniel would benefit from the basic MAC skills so that he could view his occasionally negative thoughts as a normal part of human existence and remain committed to his valued work directions. As such, and instead of avoiding, he could consistently engage in necessary daily work behaviors, even when faced with stress.

According to the case formulation model, the next step is to determine the MCS-SP classification that is most appropriate for Daniel's needs. This classification will help direct individualized intervention planning. Using the data accumulated during the assessment phase, Daniel's presenting concerns appeared to be a desire for enhanced performance. There was no evidence of significant subclinical or clinical difficulties relating to these concerns. As such, an MCS-SP classification of performance development was made (Gardner & Moore, 2004b, 2006).

INTERVENTION PLANNING AND
COURSE OF TREATMENT

The intervention plan for Daniel consisted of the seven-module MAC program. Daniel and the consultant agreed that he would receive weekly

1-hour sessions over a 7-week period. Following initial feedback and the presentation of the case formulation described earlier, Daniel and the consultant discussed and agreed to this intervention plan during his initial session. As per the basic theoretical model at the foundation of the MAC program, it was explained that the intervention would not seek or require the elimination of any thoughts or feelings, but rather would focus on the development of enhanced awareness whereby the presence of thoughts and feelings would be noted, observed, and simply allowed to exist. In addition, the consultant stressed that the overarching goal of the MAC program was the enhancement of behaviors necessary for optimal performance. Daniel suggested that the presentation was clear and was eager to get to work. He also noted that the consultant did not mention anything about him that had to be fundamentally changed or eliminated. On the contrary, the consultant described only things that needed to be *added*. This was something that Daniel felt very positive about, because it was the only reservation that he had prior to contacting the consultant.

SESSION 1: PSYCHOEDUCATION

The outline of Module 1 of the MAC program was previously identified as:

1. Introduction
2. Present the Theoretical Rationale for the MAC Program
3. Connect the Rationale to the Client's Personal Performance Experience
4. Explain Automated Self-Regulation of Elite Performance
5. Define Specific Goals of the MAC Training Program
6. Introduce the Brief Centering Exercise

Because Daniel and the consultant had met once before to conduct assessments and the initial interview, the first MAC session began with a discussion of the rationale and purpose of MAC training. Of particular importance was a discussion of the concept of self-regulation and elite performance. Daniel and the consultant discussed both functional and dysfunctional performance as presented in chapter 1, and special attention was given to the role of approach versus avoidance behavior in optimal performance. The concept that thoughts are simply thoughts and do not necessarily need to direct one's behavior was discussed in some detail. Daniel appeared to be attentive, was pleasant and interested in these concepts, and easily grasped the information presented. When it was clear that Daniel understood the model, the consultant asked him to complete the Performance Rating Form (see Figure 12.1).

Initials: DR   Date: XXXX   Age: 37   Occupation: Executive   Gender: Male

Please list performance barriers that have occurred within the last 2 weeks (such as negative thoughts, negative emotions, interpersonal problems, lack of concentration, etc.).

Putting off necessary tasks. Unwillingness to deal with the negative reaction of subordinates when giving negative feedback. Belief that I'm really not good enough and it's only a matter of time before those above me figure it out.

0	1	2	3	4	5	6	7	8
None		Mild		Moderate		Strong		Extreme

Please rate each of the following using the 0–8 scale above:

Performance Domain	Satisfaction With Performance	Impact of Performance Barrier
Preparation	8	2
Daily Work Tasks	5	8
Relationships With Staff	7	5
Relationships With Coworkers/Subordinates	5	8
Other (please describe): Home life	4	9

FIGURE 12.1   Daniel's Performance Rating Form

The information contained on Daniel's Performance Rating Form indicated that Daniel believed that barriers were negatively affecting his performance at both work and home. It was also clear that the barriers Daniel noted were consistent with the case formulation presented earlier.

At this time, Daniel and the consultant spent several minutes reviewing his goals for seeking this service and engaged in a discussion regarding the match between his goals and the primary goals of the MAC program. While Daniel reiterated his desire to improve the skills that would be needed to attain greater corporate success, he also noted his desire to learn to work in a way that would not translate into preoccupation at home and a reduced ability to be a "loving and involved husband." We discussed that the MAC's focus was on *behavior* change and not *thinking* or *feeling* change. The MAC core skill of willingness to experience "negative" thoughts and feelings in the service of what matters was also discussed. Specifically, the consultant and Daniel agreed to work on activating necessary behaviors currently being avoided, develop the ability to be aware of one's internal processes without attempting to eliminate or reduce them, and develop the ability to view one's thoughts as events that come and go and do not require attention. It was suggested that these specific enhancements would lead to more effective work behavior and a more active and involved home life. Through this dialogue, it became clear that Daniel's goals and the goals of the MAC program were highly complementary.

The Brief Centering Exercise was then presented. The goal of the exercise was carefully described as the first step in developing greater self-awareness and greater capacity to regulate his focus of attention onto the immediate moment. Importantly, the consultant also stated that the use of the Brief Centering Exercise and all similar exercises to be presented in the future are not intended to help him relax or otherwise avoid the stress of his day, but rather are implemented to help him focus on that which needs attention. Following completion of the Brief Centering Exercise, Daniel was given the Preparing for MAC handout and the What I Have Learned Form. These were to be read and completed (respectively) as soon as possible after the first MAC session. Daniel was also asked to practice the Brief Centering Exercise at least daily during the next week.

SESSION 2: MINDFULNESS AND COGNITIVE DEFUSION

The outline of Module 2 of the MAC program was previously identified as:

1. Brief Centering Exercise
2. Discussion of the What I Have Learned Form

3. Check for and Respond to Questions or Uncertainties Regarding the Previous Session
4. Rationale and Importance of Mindfulness
5. Discussion of Between-Session Exercises: What I Have Learned Form, Brief Centering Exercise, and Washing a Dish Mindfulness Exercise
6. Review Session
7. Brief Centering Exercise

Session 2 began with a Brief Centering Exercise (BCE) and continued with a discussion of Daniel's experience with the between-session use of the BCE. Daniel had done the exercise twice during the week, explaining that a particularly busy week interfered with his expectation of practicing it daily. When asked how he could possibly not have time to complete an exercise that required 3 to 5 minutes to complete, Daniel immediately became nonaggressively defensive but stopped himself in midsentence and agreed that, while he had many opportunities to practice it, he instead chose other things to do. This initiated a discussion about how the MAC program would and would not work. The consultant stated that it would be better if Daniel chose to begin the program at a later point when he was fully committed, rather than beginning at a time when he would not be willing or able to give maximum effort. Daniel insisted that he was ready for the program. The consultant remarked about the clear disconnect between the client's words and actions. Daniel agreed, and a discussion evolved concerning how the avoidant behavior responsible for noncompletion of the between-session assignment was exactly the same type of behavior that he had previously described as an impediment to full work success. It was particularly important that we address this behavioral pattern early in the MAC program due to its clear relevance. Although Daniel was clearly uncomfortable during this discussion, he indicated that he understood. He then promised that he would push through any future desires to "put it off until later" and simply practice the assignments at defined times in the day.

Following this initial discussion, the consultant inquired about the completion of the What I Have Learned Form, and, Daniel had also failed to complete this form. However, after restating his commitment to complete this and all other forms and exercises in the future, Daniel did describe in accurate detail what he had learned the week before. Daniel was able to identify the basic purpose of the MAC, the goals, his own case conceptualization, and the essential elements of optimal performance and the ways in which his recent behavior was self-defeating. Interestingly, he used his nonadherence to between-session tasks as an example of avoidance and made a concerted effort to be fully engaged in the session.

The concepts of mindfulness and cognitive defusion were then introduced. First, Daniel was asked to complete the Mindfulness Attention Awareness Scale (MAAS; Brown & Ryan, 2003), which indicated marginal mindful attention and awareness. It was explained that this instrument was to be used as a baseline of mindfulness skills and would objectively note any improvements in mindfulness during the course of the MAC program. His score on the MAAS suggested relatively low levels of mindful awareness and attention. Mindfulness was described as a central component of optimal performance through its promotion of enhanced awareness and attention, concepts that were then discussed in some detail. In this same context, cognitive defusion was presented to Daniel as the capacity to recognize that a thought is nothing more than a thought and not an absolute reflection of reality that therefore requires a specific action. Daniel understood and was able to provide personal examples of how this could help him stay focused on the tasks that needed to be completed each day. In fact, Daniel stated that becoming more mindful before the beginning of important meetings (such as executive council meetings) could very well result in better personal performance.

Next, an additional between-session assignment (the Washing a Dish Exercise) was presented, and Daniel was asked to complete the assignment three or four times during the coming week. It was stressed that this exercise was in addition to the BCE discussed earlier. The Washing a Dish Exercise was introduced as a means of further developing mindfulness skills. This exercise includes an external physical task, with instructions to focus on the various sensory experiences that naturally occur during the exercise. At the same time, the client is asked to become aware of the wide range of internal experiences such as thoughts and feelings that arise during the exercise. Daniel was asked to note these internal sensations, observe them, and then gently refocus his attention onto the washing of the dish. The goal of the exercise was presented as the simple completion of the exercise while simultaneously becoming aware of all aspects of the experience. Daniel was asked to note how easy or difficult it was to do, where his mind traveled, and what impact his thoughts had on completing the task. Daniel was also given the What I Have Learned Form to fill out after the session.

SESSION 3: INTRODUCING VALUES AND VALUES-DRIVEN BEHAVIOR

The outline of Module 3 of the MAC program was previously identified as:

1. Brief Centering Exercise
2. Discussion of the What I Have Learned Form

3. Check for and Respond to Questions or Uncertainties Regarding the Previous Session
4. Discussion and Exploration of Values and Values-Driven Versus Emotion-Driven Behavior
5. Additional Home Mindfulness Exercise: Relevant Mindful Activity
6. Discussion of Between-Session Exercises: What I Have Learned Form, Performance Values Form, Given Up for Emotions Form, and Mindfulness Exercises
7. Introduction to Mindfulness of the Breath Exercise

Session 3 began with a BCE and a discussion of the between-session practice of this exercise. Daniel indicated that he practiced the BCE every day. However, rather than doing it during a set time period, he allowed himself to be more flexible and practiced it at various times of the day, such as when he was feeling like avoiding a task that needed to be done. He reported finding that the BCE allowed him to notice and observe the thoughts that were getting in the way of completing his tasks. He also suggested that he was generally able to allow his thoughts to pass and was able to move on to the task at hand. Interestingly, he reported that, on two occasions, he used the exercise at home when thoughts about things he did or didn't do at work were becoming a preoccupation. He further indicated that, following the BCE, he was able to recognize what he needed to get done at work the next day, let go of the repetitive thoughts (which also tended to be somewhat self-damning), and then fully interact with his wife.

Following the BCE practice and discussion, our conversation moved on to the What I Have Learned Form, which Daniel also fully completed. As expected, Daniel reported in detail the information that he gleaned from the previous session and indicated a number of personal references to its relevance and accuracy. He clearly made a full effort to fulfill the promise of total investment in the program that he made the week before, and the consultant told him (honestly) that the form was completed with as much effort as he had ever seen. The consultant followed up on this successfully completed form with a brief period of time dedicated to answering questions about the material covered so far in the MAC program. Daniel did not express any questions, and it was therefore determined that the next portion of session 3 could be addressed.

The discussion of values began by presenting the distinction between goals and values. Again, Daniel had little difficulty understanding these concepts and readily began to connect values and the goals associated with values. As is customary at this point in the MAC program, the consultant presented the cross-country travel metaphor described in detail in chapter 6. Daniel was then asked to complete the Performance Obituary (see Figure 12.2), also described in chapter 6.

It became clear from reading Daniel's Performance Obituary that he identified fundamental values that he hoped could and would define him as both a husband and performer in the workplace. It was also obvious that a number of the issues that Daniel presented as the reason for seeking consultation involved behaviors that were not only problematic from the perspective of successful performance, but also from the perspective of being the person he stated a desire to be.

Consequently, it seemed appropriate for the discussion to naturally move to the difference between behaviors in the service of these values and those that are in the service of immediate emotional relief. Within this context, Daniel was able to readily note that each and every difficulty that he presented as problematic evolved directly from behavior intended to in some way reduce or prevent a variety of emotions. For instance, he was readily able to see that his avoidance of difficult conversations was a behavior in the service of prevention of personal discomfort. He was similarly able to recognize that his reluctance to check e-mail and telephone messages and his extended lunches were also in the service of prevention of personal distress, and neither was in the service of any of the performance and personal values that he defined in his Performance Obituary. Finally, Daniel was able to recognize that his behavior at home was also not in the service of a core value, and his work-related rumination at home was an effort to make himself feel better about not doing what he needed to do at the office.

At this point in session 3, Daniel was presented with the Given Up for Emotions Form and was asked to complete it before the next session. In addition, he was given the Performance Values form, which was described as a vehicle by which he could further clarify his performance values.

The session then evolved to a discussion of Daniel's experience with the Washing a Dish mindfulness exercise. Daniel indicated that he had performed the exercise three times, once in the morning before work and twice at night before bedtime. He indicated that the first time he was very distracted during the exercise and was only able to think about the upcoming workday. During this first experience, he reported great difficulty focusing on the sensations that were being experienced as he washed the dish. Like many clients completing this exercise for the first time, he also pointed out that he became frustrated while performing this exercise. The consultant noted that the exercise was effective in that Daniel noticed these reactions and was able to describe these experiences in some detail. Ultimately, this is a major goal of mindfulness exercises. Daniel also reported that he found it increasingly easy to alternate be-

Initials: DR   Date: XXXX   Age: 37   Occupation: Executive   Gender: Male

What and how would you like your performance/work career
and you as an athlete, attorney, salesperson, coworker,
teammate, etc. to be remembered?

Daniel was a dedicated family man who always made his wife

feel that she was the most important person in the world. At work

he was known as a responsible and ethical person who worked

hard, worked well, and did the right thing for his customers, his

employees, and his shareholders.

FIGURE 12.2   Daniel's Performance Obituary

tween being aware of the external sensations and the internal experiences (thoughts) that he was having each time he performed the exercise. We discussed how his reactions were very typical, and connected his choice to continue with the exercise, despite feeling frustrated and distracted, as a perfect example of an action in the service of his values and not the immediate emotion. This was contrasted to the choices that he reported frequently making at work. Another between-session mindfulness exercise was assigned and agreed upon. This exercise was comprised of mindful eating, which meant that the client should do nothing else while eating and simply notice and observe all of the sensations involved in eating. Such sensations included smell, taste, and other physical sensations. Daniel was also introduced to the Mindfulness of the Breath Exercise at this time, which was then practiced directly in-session. He was instructed to practice the Mindfulness of the Breath Exercise as well as the previously learned Brief Centering Exercise in a variety of situations during the upcoming week.

SESSION 4: INTRODUCING ACCEPTANCE AS AN ALTERNATIVE TO CONTROL

The outline of Module 4 of the MAC program was previously identified as:

1. In-Session Mindfulness Practice
2. Discuss the What I Have Learned Form, Check for and Respond to Questions or Uncertainties Regarding the Previous Session, and Discuss Reactions to the Relevant Mindful Activity Exercise
3. Review the Performance Values Form and Given Up for Emotions Form and Pursue Discussion of Obvious and Subtle Avoidance Strategies
4. Experiential Acceptance as an Alternative to Avoidance and the Connection Between Willingness and Values-Driven Committed Behavior
5. Extending the Relevant Mindful Activity Exercise
6. Brief Centering Exercise

Session 4 began with the Brief Centering Exercise and a discussion regarding its between-session use. Daniel indicated that he had successfully used the BCE daily, at home before going to work, during the workday, and once upon arriving home before interacting with his wife. He indicated that the use of this exercise had become much easier. He suggested that it was allowing him to notice and let go of his thoughts, even the ones relating to competence, thus promoting better attention to whatever it was that needed to be done. Additionally, Daniel again completed the What I Have Learned Form, which indicated that the material from the previous week was adequately understood. We moved on to a review of the Performance Values Form (see Figure 12.3), which Daniel said he completed the night after our last session.

A review of this form led to some clear conclusions. First, Daniel acknowledged that he did not complete the technical or tactical skills portions of the form, because he thought that they were already discussed and considered. The consultant chose to not address that issue, because it was apparent from the rest of the completed form that Daniel was putting forth an honest effort to complete the form in a manner that correctly identified his primary needs and issues. Second, it was apparent that Daniel was developing a clear awareness that the items he valued were not consistently pursued, not because they did not matter, but rather because of an immediate desire to feel better and/or avoid feeling bad in the first place. Third, Daniel was able to see that in each area that was designated as a value, greater effort (commitment) was required. Fourth, Daniel was able to see that sometimes a specific goal could be attained through the pursuit of values. For example, he clearly established a value of enjoyment of his work experience and recognized that, by enhancing specific skills, his enjoyment of work would likely increase. Fifth, he recognized that his personal values were just as meaningful and not in any way less meaningful than his work values. Following this discussion, we moved on to the final form completed between sessions, which was the Given Up for Emotions Form (see Figure 12.4).

A review of Daniel's form confirmed the information that we had already collected—that short-term relief was the motivating factor for the behaviors that he listed. Daniel noted that he stopped himself from the "excuse" call, and believed that becoming more self-aware was the reason. He said that, during the week, he began to feel sad when he thought about how often he avoided simple tasks simply for the purpose of feeling better at that moment. He added that he not only didn't make the excuse call to his brother-in-law, but he called to apologize and called his wife to apologize to her also. In the discussion that followed, Daniel seemed very subdued as he talked about the myriad of ways that these small avoidance behaviors manifest themselves. He suggested that if he had become so successful *with* this behavioral pattern, he might have done even better and been even happier if he had previously been able to more aggressively pursue the values he truly desired.

The session moved to a discussion of the concept of poise and its relationship to optimal performance as a senior business executive. During the conversation, Daniel indicated that he was thinking about a number of senior executives who he had met and worked with and realized that

Performance Values Form

Initials: DR   Date: XXXX   Age: 37   Occupation: Executive   Gender: Male

The following is a list of performance values that may help direct your actions on a daily basis. After each value is recorded, please identify the barriers to, and the actions that must be taken in pursuit of, those values.

Teammate/coworker: What type of teammate/coworker do you want to be? What does it mean to be a good teammate/coworker? Why is being a solid team member/coworker important to you?
Responsible. Available and concerned about the welfare of my colleagues. Teams can't be successful without the total commitment of all their members. That total commitment must come from me if I expect others to do the same.

Barriers and Necessary Actions:
Becoming overly preoccupied with my needs, especially when I don't do what's required for the larger good of the company out of concern that I will be uncomfortable facing the discomfort of an individual team member. I need to do what is necessary but difficult on a consistent basis.

Sport/Work/Performance Activity: What do you value about your activity? The challenge? Prestige? Enjoyment? Getting to interact with teammates? Helping people?
I enjoy my work, I get great satisfaction from the success of my department, and I enjoy the compensation and lifestyle that comes with my work.

Barriers and Necessary Actions:
I sometimes overreact to my stress and look for ways to be comfortable. I have to develop the attitude that comfort and success are not necessarily related.

FIGURE 12.3   Daniel's Performance Values Form

Training: Is developing your skill important to you? Why is working at getting better meaningful to you? Are there any skills you'd like to learn or develop more fully?

I know that I have to improve my financial management skills to an even higher level. This would help me enjoy my work more as well as becoming more central to the operation of my company.

Barriers and Necessary Actions:
Sometimes it seems like too much work to enhance these skills. It seems easier to do what I do best and take advantage of my other skills. I have to make this personal development a priority.

Technical Skills: What issues or behaviors related to technical skill development do you care about (e.g., time spent working on golf swing, sales presentation skills, etc.)? What would you like to do more of?

Barriers and Necessary Actions:

Tactical Skills: What issues or behaviors related to tactical skill development do you care about (e.g., effort spent on planning a sales or presentation strategy, developing greater understanding of pitch or club selection, situational play, etc.)? What would you like to do more of?

Barriers and Necessary Actions:

Recreation/Fun: What type of activities do you enjoy? Why do you enjoy them?
I enjoy my time at home with my wife. I enjoy my workout time. I enjoy our friends.

Barriers and Necessary Actions:
I don't always allow myself to throw myself into my home life because I don't feel like I've earned it. If these things matter to me, I owe it to myself to put out maximum effort at enjoying them.

FIGURE 12.3   Continued.

Given Up for Emotions Form

Initials: DR   Date: XXXX   Age: 37   Occupation: Executive   Gender: Male

The purpose of this form is to help you become more aware of what you have given up to reduce or eliminate your emotions. What opportunities in the service of your values are you giving up in the service of feeling less emotion? How is this affecting your ability to perform better and enjoy your competitive/work world more?

In the first (far left) column, list a situation related to practice, training, or actual competition/work that triggered a strong emotion. In the second column, write down the specific emotion that was experienced. In the third column, record what you did to reduce or satisfy your emotion. In the fourth column, write down what your effect efforts to control or reduce your emotion had on you. In last (far right) column, write down the long-term consequences of your efforts to rid yourself of these emotions (what you gave up to reduce or satisfy your emotion).

Complete form below:

Situation or event	Emotion	What you did to control emotion	Short-term effect	Long-term effect on you
Tell an employee that his compensation was to be cut	Anxious	Put it off for 3 weeks	Felt relieved	Increasingly uncomfortable because it had to be done
Prepare a presentation for the executive council	Anxious	Put it off until the night before	Felt relief	Increased fear and concern about how well it would be done
Forgot about brother-in-law's birthday	Frustrated and sad	Began to call him with an excuse	Would have felt some relief	Would have felt guilty

FIGURE 12.4   Daniel's Given Up for Emotions Form

one common characteristic among all of them was their ability to function at a high level regardless of what was going on around them. He concluded that they must have experienced a wide variety of emotions during the time he had observed them at work, but their behaviors were not reflective of emotionality. Rather, they "kept their eye on the ball" regardless of what they may have been feeling. Daniel noted that this was certainly an area in which he needed a great deal of work and suggested that this concept, while related to everything else that had been discussed to date, was by far the most meaningful issue to him and resonated the most with his personal style. The consultant then went on to discuss the obstacles to poise, which were primarily linked to experiential avoidance, or the desire to act in the service of immediate thoughts and feelings and not in the service of values and goals emanating from those values. This naturally led to a beneficial conversation about how emotions, no matter which ones they are and no matter how strongly they are felt, and thoughts, no matter how real they may seem or how ruminative they may be, do not directly *cause* behavior that interferes with optimal functioning. Rather, it became clear within this discussion that it is how individuals *respond* to their emotions and thoughts that determines performance outcomes. The consultant then presented Daniel with a fundamental goal of the MAC program, which was to change the frequently used statement, "I want to perform better, *but* I feel so bad," to "I want to perform better, *and* I feel so bad." Again, the consultant noted that this concept is analogous to the definition of poise and reiterated that ultimately the top performer must develop a *willingness* to remain in contact with—that is *accept*—difficult or painful internal experiences in the *committed* pursuit of performance and life *values*. Daniel easily understood the concepts, and the examples he presented in the session conveyed the idea that the concept was resulting in serious self-reflection.

The session then focused on relevant mindful exercises. Although Daniel did not perform these exercises during any preplanned performance-related moments, he had begun to use the exercises at various times of the workday. In addition, and as promised, he spent three meals each day eating mindfully. Daniel described this experience as interesting, in that as he ate one lunch mindfully, he became aware of how much he disliked the taste of carrots. He had never realized this before, which he suggested was because he typically ate very quickly and while doing other things. He also noted that he became much more aware of his eating speed and was now able to notice the food, eat more slowly, eat less, and walk away believing that he actually "experienced" a meal. The consultant noted that Daniel was now seeing the distinction between *having* a life experience and mindfully *living* a life experience, and wondered how many other areas in life he did not fully experience.

This was followed by continued discussion of relevant mindful exercises, including preplanning to mindfully converse with subordinates and to interact with them more completely and the use of the BCE at natural breaks in meetings or other business-related activities. Daniel agreed to engage in these activities, and the session ended with a BCE.

SESSION 5: ENHANCING COMMITMENT

The outline of Module 5 of the MAC program was previously identified as:

1. In-Session Mindfulness Practice
2. Review of Previous Session
3. Enhancing Commitment: Connecting Values, Goals, and Behaviors
4. Review and Assign Performance-Relevant Mindfulness Homework
5. Session Review and Brief Centering Exercise

Module 5 began with a Mindfulness of the Breath Exercise and moved to a brief review of the previous session. Daniel appeared to not only remember the content and take home the message of the previous session, but also indicated that it was "inspiring" and moved him to really think about how he conducts himself at work and at home. He volunteered to share his Emotion and Performance Interference Form (see Figure 12.5). He indicated that his completed form demonstrated how much the previous session had meant to him; he had recorded one meaningful incident and noted how he would have acted in the past and how he did act during the past week.

With this clear demonstration that Daniel both understood and had begun to act on the avoidance at the core of his presenting issues, the consultant highlighted the relationship between goals and values, and in turn how goals may occur within the context of values. Daniel easily understood the distinction between values and goals, and thus the consultant gently directed the discussion to a consideration of what day-to-day behaviors would be essential in the pursuit of his values (while also noting that they would inevitably also result in goal attainment). Daniel accurately noted that only through activating these behaviors consistently and regularly would he really show his commitment to his values. Both parties then defined these specific behaviors, which were identified as follows:

1. Responding to e-mail and telephone messages promptly (within 24 hours).

Emotion and Performance Interference Form

Initials: DR   Date: XXXX   Age: 37   Occupation: Executive   Gender: Male

Please record performance situations that occurred during the past week, the emotion(s) experienced, the degree to which these emotions interfered with performance, and how these emotions interfered with performance.

Situation	Emotion Rate Intensity 0 = none 10 = extreme	Performance Interference Rate Intensity 0 = none 10 = extreme	What Happened?

I needed to tell a long-time salesperson that she was not getting a desired and expected promotion. Felt anxiety = 7. In the past this would have led to a number of reasons to put off and dread taking this meeting, so Performance Interference = 5. Instead, I set up the meeting for the same day, and despite feeling very uncomfortable, had the meeting, gave the bad news, and allowed her to become very angry without responding in a defensive or hostile manner. So, Performance Interference = 1.

FIGURE 12.5   Daniel's Emotion and Performance Interference Form

2. Arranging and/or completing necessary meetings that involved the presentation of bad or difficult news to another employee promptly upon finding out about its necessity.
3. Asserting thoughts and opinions at executive council meetings regardless of insecure thoughts or anxious feelings.
4. Having my head and body in the same place and at the same time. Being at work when I am at work and being at home when I am at home.

While the first three of these behaviors were predictable and consistent given Daniel's presenting issues and the content of previous sessions, the last behavior was interesting in its clear connection to the definition of mindfulness. Daniel was taken by, and increasingly appreciating the degree to which, as he noted, "my body is one place but my head is somewhere else." His final specific behavior in need of activation reflected a desire to focus on the daily expression of mindful behavior at work and at home.

Daniel was asked to write down this list of behaviors and put a check next to them on every day that he successfully completed them. He was also given the Committing to Performance Values Exercise and asked to complete this form between sessions. This dialogue culminated with a review of the need to allow oneself to be willing to experience negative thoughts and emotions while actively engaging in these value-driven behaviors.

Session 5 ended with a BCE and a review of the places and times at which mindfulness was being practiced. Daniel reported using these skills and practicing his exercises in the gym, at breaks in meetings (as he previously indicated he would), when he first arrived at work, and when he arrived home in the evening. He was pleased with the value of these exercises and noted that he was becoming much more aware of yet much less affected by his thoughts and feelings at any given moment.

SESSION 6: SKILL CONSOLIDATION AND POISE: COMBINING MINDFULNESS, ACCEPTANCE, AND COMMITMENT

The outline of Module 6 of the MAC program was previously identified as:

1. In-Session Mindfulness Exercises
2. Review of Previous Session
3. Putting It All Together: Enhancing Poise Through Exposure-Based Activities

4. Review and Assign Performance-Relevant Mindfulness and Task-Focused Attention Exercises
5. Brief Centering Exercise and Review of Between-Session Forms

Module 6 began with a BCE, after which Daniel took the opportunity to express how well the mindfulness exercises were working for him. In his view, they were allowing for better self-awareness, better attention to tasks in which he was engaged, and a greater sense of personal well-being. He indicated that his mind felt more at ease and that he was more responsive to the demands of his day. Daniel also stated that his wife had remarked (without being questioned) that he was substantially more attentive to her at home, was listening better, and was a much "better person" with whom to live. From Daniel's perspective, this was ultimately the most important sign of performance enhancement, and he indicated that, while he believed he was performing more effectively and consistently at work, there was no single work-related indicator that could or should compare with his wife's comments to him.

This was followed by a discussion of his between-session exercises, at which time Daniel presented his Committing to Performance Values Exercise (see Figure 12.6). Daniel used a specific experience with his wife as an example but indicated that he had been following the same basic approach to life. In fact, he had successfully activated each behavior listed during the previous session.

The consultant took the opportunity to discuss two new items with Daniel at this time. The first was the Task-Focused Attention Exercise. This form and the purpose of the exercise were explained in detail. However, Daniel expressed a preference to remain focused on his mindfulness practice and did not see the need for this extension. Of course, the MAC program is intended to be flexible and the professional practice of psychology must always seek to incorporate the needs and preferences of the client where appropriate. However, before allowing the client to skip a valuable exercise, it should first be determined whether the client's desire is a form of experiential avoidance. In this particular case, the consultant did not see this as a form of avoidance and therefore supported Daniel's request to remain committed to the mindfulness practice. However, he stated that if Daniel became interested in greater task-focused attention in the future, it would not be a difficult add-on for someone as committed to mindfulness practice as Daniel appeared to be. Because the end of the next session would mark the formal end of the MAC protocol, the second item discussed pertained to the termination of services. Daniel indicated that he had already thought about the upcoming termination since the MAC program had previously been described as a seven-session sequence. Daniel believed that he would be able to successfully continue integrating MAC

Committing to Performance Values Exercise

Initials: DR   Date: XXXX   Age: 37   Occupation: Executive   Gender: Male

Performance Value (PV):
Being a committed husband who is totally engaged with my family.

Short-Term Goal Associated With PV:
Having more satisfying experiences with my wife.

Long-Term Goal Associated With PV:
Having a mutually satisfying long-term relationship.

Behavior To Be Added or Changed To Achieve PV:
Having fully connected conversations with my wife every evening.

Situation:
Came home at night and had dinner with my wife.

Action Taken:
Spent time asking about her day, being mindful of her conversation, and really listening to her answers.

FIGURE 12.6   Daniel's Committing to Performance Values Exercise

skills on his own, but he also wanted to be sure that he could continue in the future if he needed a "tune-up" or even more lengthy meetings. When he was assured that he could certainly see the consultant again if needed, both parties agreed to end the formal program after the seventh session and moved on to completing the remainder of Module 6.

We discussed the importance of confronting the most difficult or emotionally charged situations at work and learning to remain in those situations until the emotion abated or until able to function in the manner that was required (exposure). The consultant inquired about any remaining situations that Daniel may have been avoiding. Despite all efforts to probe for and consider a variety of possible situations, Daniel suggested that, while he could not say that he never avoided at all, he did indicate that there were really no emotional situations in which he could honestly say that he was consistently avoiding. Daniel stated that he understood the basic premise of exposure and could relate to its usefulness based on his recent success in confronting rather than avoiding difficult and uncomfortable situations. He reported that, in these situations, his anxiety had diminished over time as he remained in these situations until completed. It was clear that as a relatively healthy individual (hence his earlier performance development classification), Daniel did not have the need for the more clinically relevant variant of prolonged exposure.

The Brief Centering Exercise was completed, and an appointment was scheduled at a 3-week interval rather than the usual 1-week interval to ensure that Daniel would be able to continue his progress and engage the various exercises and principles that had been discussed during the first six modules of the MAC program.

SESSION 7: MAINTAINING AND ENHANCING MINDFULNESS-ACCEPTANCE-COMMITMENT

The outline of Module 7 of the MAC program was previously identified as:

1. Review Previous Session and Overall MAC Program
2. Brief Centering Exercise
3. Task-Focused Attention Exercise
4. Review of Current Level of Experiential Acceptance, Willingness, and Commitment to Values
5. Plan for Future Practice: Self-Reflection and Self-Correction

The final module of the MAC program began with the Brief Centering Exercise. Afterward, Daniel and the consultant spent a brief time reviewing both the previous session and the entire MAC program experience.

Performance Rating Form: Session 1

Performance Domain	Satisfaction With Performance	Impact of Performance Barriers
Preparation	8	2
Daily Work Tasks	5	8
Relationships With Staff	7	5
Relationships With Coworkers/Subordinates	5	8
Other (please describe): <u>Home Life</u>	4	9

Performance Rating Form: Session 7

Performance Domain	Satisfaction With Performance	Impact of Performance Barriers
Preparation	10	1
Daily Work Tasks	9	2
Relationships With Staff	10	2
Relationships With Coworkers/Subordinates	9	2
Other (please describe): <u>Home Life</u>	10+	1

FIGURE 12.7   Daniel's Performance Rating Form: Comparative Results From Session 1 and Session 7

Daniel stated that he could not have been happier with the results of the program and indicated that he had been more energetic, happier at work, and substantially more productive. Most importantly, this has occurred in addition to significant enhancement in what he described as an already strong marriage. He also reported that, during the previous 3 weeks (since the last session), he had continued to do all of the things that he had previously worked on, and all components were still being incorporated nicely. Following this review, Daniel was asked to again complete the Performance Rating Form. The comparison between session one and seven is noted in Figure 12.7.

Daniel rated his performance as substantially improved in every area and, importantly, rated the impact that his previously identified performance barriers continue to have as negligible. Maybe most importantly, Daniel clearly articulated that he had noticed significant improvements not only in performance outcomes, but also the psychological *processes* (i.e., enhanced awareness and attention, reduced avoidance, and enhanced behavioral activation) that are the targets of the MAC program.

The last session concluded with a review of Daniel's stated values, the specific day-to-day behaviors connected to those values, and the specific thoughts and emotions that had previously been identified as barriers. These were now identified as obstacles rather than barriers, and Daniel understood that these would realistically be present in one form or another for the rest of his life. Daniel and the consultant developed a 2-month plan to continue working on the skills learned to date, which included continued use of performance-relevant mindfulness exercises and continued use of the behavior checklist to assure adequate and consistent behavioral activation. The availability of the consultant for follow-up sessions (if needed) was reiterated. Finally, as always, the session ended with a mindfulness exercise. The final exercise was to be chosen by Daniel, and he decided to finish his MAC experience with the Mindfulness of the Breath Exercise.

CHAPTER 13

Case Study 3: Considerations in the Group Application of MAC

Throughout this book, much has been written about how to apply the MAC program to *individual* performers for the attainment of optimal performance levels and greater personal well-being. In addition, the case studies in chapters 11 and 12 highlighted the entire session-by-session MAC protocol with two clients.

Yet, when consulting as a performance psychologist, whether in business settings, athletics, the performing arts, or in other group-oriented settings, the MAC program can be effectively provided to groups or teams that desire progress for individual members *and* the greater organizational system.

We have made an effort thus far to describe some of the nuances involved in working with groups, but it will be helpful to provide a group-based case description that speaks to the common issues and challenges that accompany the group application of the MAC program.

DESCRIPTION OF THE GROUP

The MAC was utilized with 10 members of a men's professional lacrosse league team. The consultant had been retained by management to provide psychological services to the team. Following a lengthy presentation to the entire team during training camp, 10 players volunteered to participate in the seven-module protocol. Based on time constraints and the availability

259

of the team, the protocol was not afforded a flexible meeting schedule. Instead, the program consisted of seven predetermined and set meetings, one meeting per week, for 90 minutes per meeting. These meetings occurred on days of the week predetermined by the coaching staff and were on practice days that consisted of strength/conditioning work only. The players participating in the group ranged in age from 22 to 32, and the composition of the group reflected both rookies and long-time veterans of professional lacrosse and consisted of eight White and two African American athletes.

The weekly group-based MAC program was presented as being open to any and all members of the team, and, as stated, 10 players volunteered to participate. Two other team members requested individual consultation for personal issues and chose to emphasize these individual (MAC-based) contacts instead of participating in the group program. An additional 10 members of the team chose not to participate in the MAC program at this point. However, by the end of the season, all but two team members sought consultation for either personal or performance-related concerns.

The stated goal of the MAC program was to promote enhanced performance through the development of greater poise and concentration. The overarching goals of the group-administered MAC protocol were identical to that of the individually administered MAC program described throughout this text, and the group sessions followed the same organizational format. The program began with a pre-MAC meeting in which team members and the consultant discussed the group "rules"—that is, the voluntary nature of the program and the fact that any team member could choose to terminate personal involvement at any time (although the idea of making and sticking to a commitment similar to physical training was also discussed). Confidentiality was also discussed, and the consultant made it clear that, short of any issues that threatened the well-being of the athlete or others, all discussion in the group would be held in the strictest of confidence by the consultant. It was also stressed that the members of the group should hold the same level of confidentiality with fellow MAC participants. In essence, the players agreed, "What goes on in the meetings, stays in the meetings." For a full description of ethical issues that arise when working with high-level performers and teams and how to maintain adherence to the APA Ethics Code, see Moore (2003a).

The players were then asked to complete the Performance Classification Questionnaire (Gardner & Moore, 2006; Wolanin, 2005) (see Figure 13.1). Developed by Wolanin in 2004, the PCQ helps assess for the presence or absence of performance dysfunction (Pdy) according to the Multilevel Classification System for Sport Psychology (MCS-SP). Of the 10 members of the MAC group, three met criteria for Pdy, while the other seven received the performance development classification (see chapter 3 for a review of the MCS-SP).

Wolanin © 2005

Player's Name: _____ Date: _____

	Not at all true				Very true
1. I have performed at a higher level or more consistently in the past, but my current performance or development has been slowed, reduced, or delayed.	①	②	③	④	⑤
2. My personal standards sometimes make it difficult for me to perform as well as I could.	①	②	③	④	⑤
3. I am unable to perform well because of conflicts with people or other issues with people in my life.	①	②	③	④	⑤
4. Feelings or emotions such as anxiety, sadness, frustration, or anger prevent me from performing as well as I would like.	①	②	③	④	⑤
5. I rarely have difficulty staying focused and concentrating during a performance task.	①	②	③	④	⑤
6. Negative beliefs about myself such as pessimism or lack of confidence prevent me from performing as well as I would like.	①	②	③	④	⑤
7. My physical or technical skills are developed near or at their potential.	①	②	③	④	⑤
8. I am unable to perform well because of conflicts with coaches (bosses) or teammates (coworkers).	①	②	③	④	⑤
9. My thoughts or feelings make it difficult for me to perform well.	①	②	③	④	⑤
10. Negative events that are occurring around me or in my life make it more difficult for me to perform well.	①	②	③	④	⑤

Scoring: Add all scores (reverse score items 5 and 7). Scores less than 30 suggest an MCS-SP classification of PD. Scores 30 and above suggest an MCS-SP Classification of Pdy. Please remove scoring key prior to administration.

FIGURE 13.1   Performance Classification Questionnaire

After completing this brief self-report measure, the athletes were asked to describe their goals for the program. Interestingly, the seven members of the team who were classified as PD suggested very general goals, which could essentially be described, as one player aptly put it, as "becoming mentally stronger." On the other hand, the three athletes classified as Pdy noted more specific concerns related to worry, perfectionism, and, as one player noted, "too much stuff going on in my head about not doing good." Although none of the athletes had recently experienced any major injuries, the oldest team member did suggest that he needed to learn to "play smarter" and be more "mentally effective," because he was getting older and his physical skills were diminishing. Each member of the team was also asked to rate his own athletic performance (in this case, based on the previous season) on a scale of 1 to 10, with the highest score of 10 reflecting at least a complete match between ability and performance (and possibly a degree of overachievement), and the lowest score of 1 reflecting a level of performance completely inconsistent (in a negative way) with ability level. Overall participant scores on this brief self-report measure ranged from 3 to 7. Participants classified as having performance dysfunction generated scores of 3, 3, and 5, and the total mean rating for all participants was 5.

COMMON ISSUES WITH MAC GROUP WORK

Rather than proceeding through the MAC program session-by-session as done previously, the remainder of the chapter presents an overview of the issues and challenges that confront the consultant when utilizing the MAC in a group or team setting, and how these issues were reflected with the lacrosse team. These issues will be presented in no particular order, because the combination and sequencing of these issues will vary with every MAC group.

REVIEWING PARTICIPANTS' WEEKLY PROGRESS AND EXERCISE COMPLETION

One of the challenges to engaging in an experientially intensive program like the MAC is ensuring that all participants are both completing and receiving maximum benefit from their between-session forms and exercises. Taking time to painstakingly review each participant's forms would take nearly the entire session. Instead, we suggest that the consultant engage in a thorough discussion of the between-session exercises in a manner that gets everyone involved. The forms and exercises completed between sessions should be used as the anchor for these discussions. We have found it helpful to begin relevant discussions by asking a participant to share his or her experience with the forms and exercises. Other members will inevitably discuss their own experiences and note their effective and ineffective attempts to complete the forms and exercises. It is important to remember that the exercises and forms used in the MAC program are for the purpose of promoting understanding and skill development and are *not* an end in and of themselves. If the consultant focuses on the content of the modules and seeks to ensure that the basic ideas are understood and the correct skills are being developed, progress will occur. Although it is impossible to expect that all group members will understand the MAC concepts and develop MAC skills at the same speed, it is nevertheless imperative that the consultant make a concerted effort, especially during the early stages of MAC, to help those participants having the greatest difficulty reach the necessary level of understanding. In the group-based MAC, this is often best accomplished through a fully integrated group discussion in which each participant is asked to provide an example or provide some personal connection to the material in question. We suggest a highly experiential approach to the group-administered MAC program.

By way of example, consider the MAC lacrosse group. In the first two meetings, corresponding to MAC Modules 1 and 2, it became clear that two of the participants were very much invested in the program and were fastidious in completing their forms and exercises. Five participants were moderately invested (a more typical state of affairs) and completed the required forms with accurate but minimal amounts of information. Three group members were minimally engaged in the program; they did not complete between-session forms and did not engage in the required between-session exercises. The challenge inherent in this type of scenario is maintaining the structure and sequence of the program while determining the reason(s) for the lack of committed work. Is the reason based on a lack of understanding? A reluctance to make errors in front of teammates (which was the case with two members) or perhaps a belief that the program should not require this much work (which was the case with the third participant)? Most group efforts will be similar to this case. In such situations, the consultant needs to involve all group members in a discussion about what performance enhancement is (perhaps seen as similar to physical training) and what it takes (perhaps linked to efforts at physical training). It is also useful to have participants who did engage in the program discuss their between-session experiences, reasons for doing (and not doing) between-session activities, and present their understanding of covered material. We have found it helpful to ask engaged members (especially if they are team leaders, as was the case in this situation) to offer suggestions to the less-engaged members regarding the advantages and usefulness of the exercises. It has been our experience that athletes in particular will often "call out" teammates who make excuses for not engaging in the required tasks. If a lack of conceptual understanding is a central issue, then time must be spent addressing those concepts that are unclear or poorly understood. If the issue is one of commitment, then this issue also must be addressed.

CHOOSING WHEN TO EXTEND MODULES

Related to the issues of reviewing between-session forms and exercises, and ensuring adequate understanding of concepts for each participant, is knowing when to extend one or more of the seven MAC modules to more than one session. There are several issues involved here. The first is pragmatic. The question that needs to be answered is the degree to which the consultant and the group have such flexibility. With the lacrosse team, and in many situations involving high-level sports and performing arts, time is a precious commodity, and additional time for such structured activities is rarely available. In this case, there was no time to prolong the MAC program. In fact, it was exceedingly difficult to schedule the seven sessions that were required. In optimal situations in which there is flexibility with time, the consultant can better allow the group needs and issues to determine the length of intervention. In all cases, however, the consultant should remain faithful to the sequencing and structure of the MAC protocol and do one's best to achieve the optimal results within the time allotted.

In general, we have found that the larger the number of participants in the group who have performance dysfunction, the more likely it will be that additional sessions will be necessary to fully complete the goals of each module for the reasons noted earlier in this book. Conversely, with fewer Pdy participants, it is more likely that a seven-session format will be sufficient. It should not be assumed, though, that the MCS-SP classifications are related to the *level* of the performers. We have seen top-level professional groups with numerous Pdy participants and lower-performing groups with all PD participants.

ENSURING THAT EACH PARTICIPANT RECEIVES ADEQUATE IN-SESSION MINDFULNESS PRACTICE

Given the central place of mindfulness exercises in the MAC program, it is particularly important that sufficient time is allotted for in-session mindfulness practice. Consultants who are new to the MAC program often become overly focused on the educational/didactic aspects of the MAC program and reduce or forget to allow adequate time for in-session mindfulness exercises. This includes time for both the actual exercises and time for the post-exercise discussion about the experience. It is especially important that the group members have the opportunity to discuss their difficulties or successes in using these exercises and the relevance of these exercises to their chosen activity. For example, in the lacrosse group highlighted here, one of the most important early moments of the MAC program followed an in-session centering exercise when a group participant pointed out that the difficulty he was having in "noticing and letting go" of random thoughts in the exercise was similar to his experience with negative thoughts during games. He proceeded to point out that, during the between-session Washing a Dish exercise, he experienced difficulties when focusing on a task that he did not care for, without becoming distracted and upset. He linked this to what he faces when engaged in off-season conditioning programs. These comments resulted in a lively conversation about the role of mindfulness and the corresponding state of mind*less*ness in which they often engaged. This conversation brought the purpose of MAC into clear focus and enhanced the commitment of the entire group, including those who did not contribute much to the discussion. It is important to stress that it was only through the actual in-session mindfulness exercise that this important discussion ensued. Each session began with a mindfulness exercise, was followed with an immediate discussion about the experience of the mindfulness exercise, a review of between-session experiences regarding mindfulness exercises, and finished with another mindfulness exercise of some type. This structure made the point to all members that mindfulness practice and skill development was central to the entire MAC program.

INTEGRATING EMERGING GROUP ISSUES INTO THE MAC PROGRAM

Group issues can become part of the MAC program in either of two ways. First, personal and group issues may emerge in the context of delivering the MAC. With the lacrosse team, when one participant who did not complete a between-session exercise began to explain his reasons for not completing it, another participant interrupted and pointed out that this is the same thing he does all the time—that is, he apparently found "excuses" for not doing what he was supposed to do. This issue had been lying just under the surface between this particular athlete and a number of his teammates, and his approach to the MAC program pushed the issue to the fore. Following this unexpected revelation, the consultant focused the group on the impact that one's behavior can have on others. This can be seen in a number of ways, such as one's personal responsibility to a team or demonstrating effective leadership by appropriately verbalizing negative feedback to a teammate. With this particular athlete, the focal point was on making a personal commitment to focusing on one's own behaviors in order to determine how such behaviors needed to be modified to better fit into one's personal and team values. In this case, the issues and discussions that emerged within the MAC program prompted a preexisting conflict to emerge and thus laid the groundwork for remediation and growth.

The second way in which group issues can enter into the MAC program is when an emerging group issue enters into the MAC discussion. With the lacrosse team, new financial issues within the organization created rumors about impending trades and the possible relocation of the team. In such situations, the consultant is advised to allow a brief time for the venting of participants' thoughts and feelings, after which the consultant connects the issue in a relevant manner to the appropriate MAC theme. For example, thoughts and feelings about the financial difficulties of the team are real and unavoidable. But these difficulties can still *coexist* with each member's commitment to remaining engaged in necessary practice and preparation for the season ahead. The idea that one can have negative thoughts and feelings and can face adversity and *still* fully engage in productive activities is a critical MAC concept that can be brought to life to all MAC participants in the midst of an emerging issue or concern.

TEAM VERSUS INDIVIDUAL VALUES

When delivering the MAC to individual performers, the consultant typically focuses only on the values identified by the performer for him- or herself. However, when dealing with groups—especially athletes, executives, or military personnel—group values must be carefully considered. For example, some managers, coaches, and organizational administrators establish a value of personal sacrifice and work ethic for the betterment of the larger group, and some teams and organizations become known for these values. It is important for the consultant to determine the degree to which he or she may be responsible for the promotion and development of that larger culture. Obviously, this decision is a complex one requiring a careful consideration of the consultant's role with the organization, its management, and its individual members. In the best of all situations, individual performers' values will match those of the team or organization. In our experience, this is the most common situation. However, at times, this may not occur and the consultant must quickly and carefully weigh his or her professional responsibilities (promoting the overall organizational values or the conflicting personal values of an individual member). In addition, it can be difficult to work on promoting disparate individual values in a group format, such as when one person wants to be seen as a hard worker, one wants to be seen as a good teammate, one wants to look back on his career and know he got the most out of it, and so on. It is far more useful and pragmatic for group members to establish overarching values that they could all subscribe to and use these group-developed values as a foundation for the MAC program. Individual members can, of course, apply the MAC principles to personal values and should be encouraged to share this process with the group, but an underlying core set of values may be the helpful string that ties all group members together.

Finally, the consultant must ensure that trust and openness are established prior to engaging the group members in a discussion of values. In a group-delivered MAC program, participants are, by definition, asked to share rather personal thoughts and feelings about what is truly important to them as a part of a high-performing team. This will only happen if the participants trust each other, trust the consultant, and have been helped to see the relevance of values identification as a central component of efforts at performance enhancement.

DEALING WITH MISSED SESSIONS

As is the case with all psychological interventions, the issue of missed sessions must be addressed in the group-delivered MAC program for the welfare of each individual and the overall group. Missed sessions will inevitably place the individual client and the larger group at different developmental levels with respect to MAC knowledge and skills, and, as such, make the job of the consultant more difficult. If possible, making up a single missed session through a brief individual contact is the best option. Unfortunately, this is not always a viable option. With the lacrosse team, individual sessions were not feasible due to time limitations. So, to keep all members on track, the consultant held a brief phone consultation with the individual team member who missed the session and asked that he subsequently discuss the phone session material with a teammate of his choice. This solution worked adequately in this situation, but it is clear that this cannot be a frequent occurrence. The best option is to limit the problem through an open and direct conversation during the first MAC session regarding the critical nature of full and complete attendance. Although this generally works, there will inevitably be a missed appointment or two. The team member previously noted missed the session because of an unavoidable conflict in schedule (an MRI was needed). This is typical of the time conflicts that arise when working with high-performance groups, and other relevant scenarios can be easily recognized (such as an unexpected business trip by a group member trying to close a deal). The brief phone consultation model works well, but should have set limitations.

GROUPS WITH BOTH PD AND PDY PARTICIPANTS

An interesting challenge is the inevitable reality that many groups will be composed of some combination of performers in the performance development category and those who are experiencing performance dysfunction. Yet, as previously noted, it is likely that high-level teams will primarily consist of PD members and will have only a few individuals meeting Pdy criteria (if any). Let us begin, though, by making a clear statement that there is *no* reason to believe that Pdy clients cannot make great strides during a seven-session group-based approach. Many clients with performance dysfunction will excel and prosper right along with the PD individuals. However, for other individuals with performance dysfunction, strides will be delayed. Due to vast possible permutations, simple recommendations are difficult to make, but when a large number of Pdy participants (more than one-third of the group members) are present, we recommend one of three strategies.

The first strategy is as follows. Prior to beginning the group program, the consultant can recommend to clients with performance dysfunction that they not join the group, but instead engage only in individual sessions. This option can be chosen if: (a) the seven-session group program cannot be extended past 7 weeks; (b) the consultant can be available for individual MAC interventions; (c) the struggles of numerous Pdy participants would significantly impede the gains of other group members; and (d) limiting the number of individuals in the group with performance dysfunction would lead to greater personal benefits for each individual performer and also greater benefits for the group as they are able to proceed through the group-based program without excessive delay.

The second strategy that can be utilized when more than one-third of the group members would be Pdy clients is to run the group as though it was *fully* comprised of Pdy participants. As such, a seven-session format is unlikely to be fully effective, and this should be stressed to organizational management at the outset. This recommendation is based on our experience that a high percentage of participants with performance dysfunction in a given group will inevitably require more time for each module to be effectively completed. If the group is not adjusted accordingly, the Pdy participants are likely to become frustrated at their lack of progress, and PD group members may resent being held back. This can impact everyone's in- and out-of-session activities and can clearly result in the PD participants receiving limited benefits from the program. Thus, the consultant can run the entire group at a slower pace, but he or she must make sure that such an extension is feasible.

Regardless of the specific composition of PD and Pdy group members, the consultant should carefully assess the degree to which Pdy group participants can benefit from the seven-session MAC protocol (if it cannot be extended). In situations in which pragmatic considerations do not allow for an extension of the number of MAC sessions, and when individualized MAC programs cannot be undertaken with each Pdy participant, the third option is to recommend additional individual sessions to Pdy members *following* the completion of the seven-session group protocol. Following the completion of the MAC program, all participants have brief individual summary meetings. These can take as little as 5 to 10 minutes to complete and typically include a summary of the material covered, outcome results (if available), and a reminder of the ongoing plan for the use of MAC going forward. The entire seven-session group protocol can be administered as planned, with specific attention to performance dysfunction issues only when necessary. Yet, in the final summary meeting with those Pdy clients who have not achieved maximum benefit from the seven-session group format, the consultant can encourage them to continue through individual contacts. The likelihood of this occurring will depend on the setting, the role of the consultant with the group or organization, and the personal relationship developed between the client and the consultant over the course of the first 7 weeks.

To highlight this option with the lacrosse team, slightly less than one-third of the participants were classified as experiencing performance dysfunction. It was therefore decided that the seven-session group program would be run as designed (in addition, there was no viable option for additional full sessions). Although we were able to proceed with little difficulty, 2 of the 10 participants (both of whom were classified as Pdy) made only limited progress by the end of the program, while the other 8 members made substantial gains. During the post-MAC summary meetings, the consultant discussed with these 2 individuals the need for additional brief meetings to achieve maximum benefit from the program. The consultant made a point of explaining the reason, indicating that some issues that interfere with optimal performance do not neatly fit into a structured 7-week program. Because the groundwork had already been laid and these two individuals were already familiar with the MAC program and the target constructs, it was (and should be) expected that additional progress will occur quickly when more personal attention is given. One of the two individuals decided to engage in additional individual contacts, and after several intermittent contacts, he began to demonstrate some profound changes in his behavior and performance. The other individual declined additional services, but suggested that he may reinitiate contact in the future.

FINAL GROUP SUMMARY

At the completion of Module 7 of the MAC program, the consultant asked the participants to once again complete the PCQ and the performance rating scale administered at the beginning of the MAC program. At this time, only one participant still met criteria for Pdy (as assessed by the PCQ), and the self-report ratings of performance now ranged from 5 to 10, with five players rating their performance a 10, three rating themselves as an 8, one rating himself as a 7, and one rating himself as a 5. This resulted in a mean rating of 8.5, as compared to the original preintervention mean rating of 5. While certainly not intended to be a formal experimental design, the improvements in self-ratings of performance are nonetheless consistent with a recent randomized controlled trial of the MAC (discussed in chapter 2) and reflect our personal experience with the success of the MAC protocol. Importantly, the coaching staff noted the performance gains made by many of the MAC participants and indicated that participation in the MAC program would be required of all members of the team prior to the next competitive season.

References

American Psychiatric Association. (2000). *Diagnostic and statistical manual of mental disorders* (4th ed., Rev.). Washington, DC: Author.

Andersen, M. B. (2002). Helping college student-athletes in and out of sport. In J. L. Van Raalte & B. W. Brewer (Eds.), *Exploring sport and exercise psychology* (pp. 373–393). Washington, DC: American Psychological Association.

Baer, R. A. (2003). Mindfulness training as a clinical intervention: A conceptual and empirical review. *Clinical Psychology: Science and Practice, 10,* 125–143.

Baillie, P. H. F., & Ogilvie, B. C. (2002). Working with elite athletes. In J. L. Van Raalte & B. W. Brewer (Eds.), *Exploring sport and exercise psychology* (2nd ed., pp. 395–415). Washington, DC: American Psychological Association.

Barlow, D. H. (1986). Causes of sexual dysfunction: The role of anxiety and cognitive interference. *Journal of Consulting and Clinical Psychology, 54,* 140–148.

Barlow, D. H. (Ed.). (2001). *Clinical handbook of psychological disorders* (3rd ed.). New York: Guilford Press.

Barlow, D. H. (2002). *Anxiety and its disorders: The nature and treatment of anxiety and panic* (2nd ed.). New York: Guilford Press.

Barlow, D. H., Allen, L. B., & Choate, M. L. (2004). Toward a unified treatment for emotional disorders. *Behavior Therapy, 35,* 205–230.

Bauman, J. (2000, October). Toward consensus on professional training issues in sport psychology. In E. Dunlap (Chair), *Toward consensus on professional training issues in sport psychology.* Panel discussion presented at the conference for the Association for the Advancement of Applied Sport Psychology, Nashville, TN.

Beck, A. T., Emery, G., & Greenberg, L. (1985). *Anxiety disorders and phobias: A cognitive perspective.* New York: Basic Books.

Beck, A. T., Steer, R. A., & Brown, G. K. (1996). *Manual for the Beck Depression Inventory* (2nd ed.). San Antonio, TX: Psychological Corporation.

Bergman, R. L., & Craske, M. G. (1994, November). *Covert verbalization and imagery in worry activity.* Poster session presented at the annual conference of the Association for Advancement of Behavior Therapy, San Diego, CA.

Beutler, L. E., & Consoli, A. J. (1993). Matching the therapist's interpersonal stance to clients' characteristics: Contributions from systematic eclectic psychotherapy. *Psychotherapy: Theory, Research, Practice, Training, 30,* 417–422.

Beutler, L. E., Consoli, A. J., & Williams, R. E. (1995). Integrative and eclectic therapies in practice. In B. M. Bonger & L. E. Beutler (Eds.), *Comprehensive textbook of psychotherapy: Theory and practice* (pp. 274–292). London: Oxford University Press.

Blatt, S. J., Shahal, G., & Zurhoff, D. C. (2002). Anaclitic/sociotropic and introjective/autonomous dimensions. In J. C. Norcross (Ed.), *Psychotherapy relationships that work* (pp. 315–334). New York: Oxford University Press.

Bogels, S. M., Sijbers, G. F. V., & Voncken, M. (2006). Mindfulness and task concentration training for social phobics: A pilot study. *Journal of Cognitive Psychotherapy, 20*, 33–44.

Bond, F. W., & Bunce, D. (2000). Mediators of change in emotion-focused and problem-focused worksite stress management interventions. *Journal of Occupational Health Psychology, 5*, 156–163.

Bond, J. W. (2001). The provision of sport psychology services during competition tours. In G. Tenenbaum (Ed.), *The practice of sport psychology* (pp. 217–229). Morgantown, WV: Fitness Information Technology.

Borkovec, T. D. (1994). The nature, functions, and origins of worry. In G. Davey & F. Tallis (Eds.), *Worrying: Perspectives on theory, assessment, and treatment* (pp. 5–33). Sussex, England: Wiley.

Borkovec, T. D., & Inz, J. (1990). The nature of worry in generalized anxiety disorder: A predominance of thought activity. *Behaviour Research and Therapy, 28*, 153–158.

Borkovec, T. D., Lyonfields, J. D., Wiser, S. L., & Deihl, L. (1993). The role of worrisome thinking in the suppression of cardiovascular response to phobic imagery. *Behaviour Research and Therapy, 31*, 321–324.

Bouton, M. E. (1993). Context, time, and memory retrieval in the interface paradigms of Pavlovian learning. *Psychological Bulletin, 114*, 80–99.

Bouton, M. E. (2002). Context, ambiguity, and unlearning: Sources of relapse after behavioral extinction. *Biological Psychiatry, 52*, 976–986.

Brown, K. W., & Ryan, R. M. (2003). The benefits of being mindful: Mindfulness and its role in psychological well-being. *Journal of Personality and Social Psychology, 84*, 822–848.

Burke, B. L., Arkowitz, H., & Menchola, M. (2003). The efficacy of motivational interviewing: A meta-analysis of controlled clinical trials. *Journal of Consulting and Clinical Psychology, 71*, 843–861.

Burton, D., Naylor, S., & Holliday, B. (2001). Goal setting in sport: Investigating the goal effectiveness paradox. In R. N. Singer, H. A. Hausenblas, & C. M. Janelle (Eds.), *Handbook of sport psychology* (2nd ed., pp. 497–528). New York: Wiley.

Carson, J. W., Carson, K. M., Gil, K. M., & Baucom, D. H. (2004). Mindfulness-based relationship enhancement. *Behavior Therapy, 35*, 471–494.

Carter, W. R., Johnson, M. C., & Borkovec, T. D. (1986). Worry: An electrocortical analysis. *Advances in Behaviour Research and Therapy, 8*, 193–204.

Carver, C. S., & Scheier, M. F. (1988). A control perspective on anxiety. *Anxiety Research, 1*, 17–22.

Castonguay, L. G., & Beutler, L. E. (Eds.). (2006). *Principles of therapeutic change that work*. Oxford, England: Oxford University Press.

Cates, J. A. (1999). The art of assessment in psychology: Ethics, expertise, and validity. *Journal of Clinical Psychology, 55*, 631–641.

Chambless, D. L., & Hollon, S. D. (1998). Defining empirically supported therapies. *Journal of Consulting and Clinical Psychology, 66*, 7–18.

Clark, D. M., Ball, S., & Pape, K. (1991). An experimental investigation of thought suppression. *Behavior Research and Therapy, 31*, 207–210.

Cohen, A., Pargman, D., & Tenenbaum, G. (2003). Critical elaboration and empirical investigation of the cusp catastrophe model: A lesson for practitioners. *Journal of Applied Sport Psychology, 15*, 144–159.

Craft, L. L., Magyar, T. M., Becker, B. J., & Feltz, D. L. (2003). The relationship between the Competitive State Anxiety Inventory-2 and sport performance: A meta-analysis. *Journal of Sport and Exercise Psychology, 25*, 44–65.

Cranston-Cuebas, M. A., & Barlow, D. H. (1995). *Attentional focus and the misattribution of male sexual arousal.* Unpublished manuscript.

Cranston-Cuebas, M. A., Barlow, D. H., Mitchell, W. B., & Athanasiou, R. (1993). Differential effects of a misattribution manipulation on sexually functional and dysfunctional males. *Journal of Abnormal Psychology, 102,* 525–533.

Craske, M. G. (1999). *Anxiety disorders: Psychological approaches to theory and treatment.* Boulder, CO: Westview Press.

Crews, D. J., & Landers, D. M. (1993). Electroencephalographic measures of attentional patterns prior to the golf putt. *Medicine and Science in Sports and Exercise, 25,* 116–126.

Crocker, P. R. E., Alderman, R. B., & Smith, M. R. (1988). Cognitive-affective stress management training with high performance youth volleyball players: Effects on affect, cognition, and performance. *Journal of Sport and Exercise Psychology, 10,* 448–460.

Csikszentmihalyi, M. (1975). *Beyond boredom and anxiety.* San Francisco: Jossey-Bass.

Csikszentmihalyi, M. (1990). *Flow: The psychology of optimal experience.* New York: Harper & Row.

Davey, G. C. L., Hampton, J., Farrell, J., & Davidson, S. (1992). Some characteristics of worrying: Evidence for worrying and anxiety as separate constructs. *Personality and Individual Differences, 13,* 133–147.

Davidson, R. J., Kabat-Zinn, J., Schumacher, J., Rosenkranz, M., Muller, D., Santorelli, S. F., et al. (2003). Alterations in brain and immune function produced by mindfulness meditation. *Psychosomatic Medicine, 65,* 564–570.

Daw, J., & Burton, D. (1994). Evaluation of a comprehensive psychological skills training program for collegiate tennis players. *The Sport Psychologist, 8,* 37–57.

Dishman, R. K. (1983). Identity crises in North American sport psychology: Academics in professional issues. *Journal of Sport Psychology, 5,* 123–134.

Dorfman, H. A. (1990). Reflections on providing personal performance enhancement consulting services in professional baseball. *The Sport Psychologist, 4,* 341–346.

Dowd, E. T., Milne, C. R., & Wise, S. L. (1991). The therapeutic reactance scale: A measure of psychological reactance. *Journal of Counseling and Development, 69,* 541–545.

Dowd, E. T., Wallbrown, F., Sanders, D., & Yesenosky, J. M. (1994). Psychological reactance and its relationship to normal personality variables. *Cognitive Therapy and Research, 18,* 601–612.

D'Urso, V., Petrosso, A., & Robazza, C. (2002). Emotions, perceived qualities, and performance of rugby players. *The Sport Psychologist, 16,* 173–199.

Edwards, T., Kingston, K., Hardy, L., & Gould, D. (2002). A qualitative analysis of catastrophic performances and the associated thoughts, feelings, and emotions. *The Sport Psychologist, 16,* 1–19.

Eifert, G. H., & Forsyth, J. P. (2005). *Acceptance and commitment therapy for anxiety disorders.* Oakland, CA: New Harbinger Publications.

First, M. B., Spitzer, R. L., Gibbon, M., & Williams, J. B. W. (1997). *User's guide for the Structured Clinical Interview for DSM-IV Axis I Disorders-clinician version (SCID-I).* New York: New York State Psychiatric Institute.

Forsberg, L., Halldin, J., & Wennberg, P. (2003). Psychometric properties and factor structure of the Readiness for Change Questionnaire. *Alcohol and Alcoholism, 38,* 276–280.

Freeston, M. H., Dugas, M. J., & Ladouceur, R. (1996). Thoughts, images, worry, and anxiety. *Cognitive Therapy and Research, 20,* 265–273.

Frost, R. O., Marten, P., Lahart, C., & Rosenblate, R. (1990). The dimensions of perfectionism. *Cognitive Therapy and Research, 14,* 449–468.

Gardner, F. L. (1995). The coach and the team psychologist: An integrated organizational model. In S. M. Murphy (Ed.), *Sport psychology interventions* (pp. 147–175). Champaign, IL: Human Kinetics.

Gardner, F. L., & Moore, Z. E. (2001, October). *The Multi-level Classification System for Sport Psychology (MCS-SP): Toward a structured assessment and conceptualization of athlete-clients.* Workshop presented at the annual conference of the Association for the Advancement of Applied Sport Psychology, Orlando, FL.

Gardner, F. L., & Moore, Z. E. (2004a). A Mindfulness-Acceptance-Commitment based approach to performance enhancement: Theoretical considerations. *Behavior Therapy, 35,* 707–723.

Gardner, F. L., & Moore, Z. E. (2004b). The Multi-level Classification System for Sport Psychology (MCS-SP). *The Sport Psychologist, 18,* 89–109.

Gardner, F. L., & Moore, Z. E. (2005). Using a case formulation approach in sport psychology consulting. *The Sport Psychologist, 19,* 430–445.

Gardner, F. L., & Moore, Z. E. (2006). *Clinical sport psychology.* Champaign, IL: Human Kinetics.

Gardner, F. L., & Moore, Z. E. (in press). Understanding clinical anger and violence: The anger avoidance model. *Behavior Modification.*

Gardner, F. L., Wolanin, A. T., & Moore, Z. E. (2005). *Mindfulness-Acceptance-Commitment (MAC) performance enhancement for Division I collegiate athletes: A preliminary investigation.* Manuscript in preparation.

Giges, B. (2000). Removing psychological barriers: Clearing the way. In M. B. Andersen (Ed.), *Doing sport psychology* (pp. 17–32). Champaign, IL: Human Kinetics.

Gordin, R. D., & Henschen, K. P. (1989). Preparing the USA women's artistic gymnastics team for the 1988 Olympics: A multi-modal approach. *The Sport Psychologist, 3,* 366–373.

Gould, D., Damarjian, N., & Greenleaf, C. (2002). Imagery training for peak performance. In J. L. Van Raalte & B. W. Brewer (Eds.), *Exploring sport and exercise psychology* (2nd ed., pp. 49–74). Washington, DC: American Psychological Association.

Gould, D., Eklund, R. C., & Jackson, S. A. (1992). 1988 U.S. Olympic wrestling excellence: I. Mental preparation, precompetitive cognition, and affect. *The Sport Psychologist, 6,* 358–382.

Gould, D., & Udry, E. (1994). Psychological skills for enhancing performance: Arousal regulation strategies. *Medicine and Science in Sport and Exercise, 26,* 478–485.

Gould, D., Weiss, M., & Weinberg, R. (1981). Psychological characteristics of successful and nonsuccessful Big Ten wrestlers. *Journal of Sport Psychology, 3,* 69–81.

Gross, J. J., & Levenson, R. W. (1997). Hiding feelings: The acute effects of inhibiting negative and positive emotion. *Journal of Abnormal Psychology, 106,* 95–103.

Groth-Marnat, G. (1999). *Handbook of psychological assessment* (3rd ed.). New York: Wiley.

Grove, W. M., Zald, D. H., Lebow, B. S., Snitz, B. E., & Nelson, C. (2000). Clinical versus mechanical prediction: A meta-analysis. *Psychological Assessment, 12,* 19–30.

Halliwell, W. (1990). Providing sport psychology consulting services in professional hockey. *The Sport Psychologist, 4,* 369–377.

Hanin, Y. L. (1980). A study of anxiety in sport. In W. F. Straub (Ed.), *Sport psychology: An analysis of athlete behavior* (pp. 236–249). Ithaca, NY: Movement Publications.

Hardy, L., Jones, G., & Gould, D. (1996). *Understanding psychological preparation for sport: Theory and practice of elite performers.* New York: Wiley.

Harvey, A., Watkins, E., Mansell, W., & Shafran, R. (2004). *Cognitive behavioural processes across psychological disorders: A transdiagnostic approach to research and treatment.* New York: Oxford University Press.

Hatfield, B. D., Landers, D. M., & Ray, W. J. (1984). Cognitive processes during self-paced motor performance: An electroencephalographic profile of skilled marksmen. *Journal of Sport Psychology, 6,* 42–59.

Hayes, S. C., Follete, V. M., & Linehan, M. M. (Eds.). (2004). *Mindfulness and acceptance: Expanding the cognitive behavioral tradition.* New York: Guilford Press.

Hayes, S. C., Kohlenberg, B. S., & Melancon, S. M. (1989). Avoiding and altering rule-control as a strategy of clinical intervention. In S. C. Hayes (Ed.), *Rule governed behavior: Cognition, contingencies, and instructional control.* New York: Plenum.

Hayes, S. C., Strosahl, K., & Wilson, K. G. (1999). *Acceptance and commitment therapy: An experiential approach to behavior change.* New York: Guilford Press.

Hayes, S. C., Strosahl, K., Wilson, K. G., Bissett, R. T., Pistorello, J., Toarmino, D., et al. (2004). The Acceptance and Action Questionnaire (AAQ) as a measure of experiential avoidance. *Psychological Record, 54,* 553–578.

Hayes, S. C., Wilson, K. G., Gifford, E. V., Follette, V. M., & Strosahl, K. (1996). Experiential avoidance and behavioral disorders: A functional dimensional approach to diagnosis and treatment. *Journal of Consulting and Clinical Psychology, 64,* 1152–1168.

Hogan, R., Hogan, J., & Roberts, B. W. (1996). Personality measurement and employment decisions: Questions and answers. *American Psychologist, 51,* 469–477.

Holm, J. E., Beckwith, B. E., Ehde, D. M., & Tinius, T. P. (1996). Cognitive-behavioral interventions for improving performance in competitive athletes: A controlled treatment outcome study. *International Journal of Sport Psychology, 27,* 463–475.

Hopson, B., & Adams, J. (1977). Toward an understanding of termination: Defining some boundaries of termination. In J. Adams, J. Hayes, & B. Hopson (Eds.), *Transition: Understanding and managing personal change* (pp. 3–25). Montclair, NJ: Allanheld & Osmun.

Janelle, C. M., Hillman, C. H., Apparies, R. J., Murray, N. P., Meili, L., Fallon, E. A., et al. (2000). Expertise differences in cortical activation and gaze behavior during rifle shooting. *Journal of Sport and Exercise Psychology, 22,* 167–182.

Janelle, C. M., Hillman, C. H., & Hatfield, B. D. (2000). Concurrent measurement of electroencephalographic and ocular indices of attention during rifle shooting: An exploratory case study. *International Journal of Sport Vision, 6,* 21–29.

Jones, G., Hanton, S., & Swain, A. B. J. (1994). Intensity and interpretation of anxiety symptoms in elite and non-elite sports performers. *Personality and Individual Differences, 17,* 657–663.

Jones, G., Swain, A. B. J., & Hardy, L. (1993). Intensity and direction dimensions of competitive state anxiety and relationships with performance. *Journal of Sport Sciences, 11,* 525–532.

Jones, J. C., Bruce, T. J., & Barlow, D. H. (1986, November). *The effects of four levels of "anxiety" on sexual arousal in sexually functional and dysfunctional men.* Poster session presented at the annual conference of the Association for Advancement of Behavior Therapy, Chicago, IL.

Kabat-Zinn, J. (1990). *Full catastrophe living: Using the wisdom of your body and mind to face stress, pain, and illness.* New York: Delta.

Kabat-Zinn, J. (1994). *Wherever you go there you are.* New York: Hyperion.

Kabat-Zinn, J., Massion, A. O., Kristeller, J., Peterson, L. G., Fletcher, K. E., Pbert, L., et al. (1992). Effectiveness of a meditation-based stress reduction program in the treatment of anxiety disorders. *American Journal of Psychiatry, 149,* 936–943.

Kendall, P. C., & Chambless, D. L. (Eds.). (1998). Empirically supported psychological therapies [Special issue]. *Journal of Consulting and Clinical Psychology, 66.*

Klinger, E., Barta, S. G., & Glas, R. A. (1981). Thought content and gap time in basketball. *Cognitive Therapy and Research, 5,* 109–114.

Kohlenberg, R. J., & Tsai, M. (1995). Functional analytic psychotherapy: Behavioral approach to intensive treatment. In W. T. O'Donohue & L. Krasner (Eds.), *Theories of behavior therapy: Exploring behavior change* (pp. 637–658). Washington, DC: American Psychological Association.

Kubler-Ross, E. (1969). *On death and dying.* New York: Macmillan.

Lilienfeld, S. O., Lynn, S. J., & Lohr, J. M. (2003). Science and pseudoscience in clinical psychology: Initial thoughts, reflections, and considerations. In S. O. Lilienfeld, S. J. Lynn, & J. M. Lohr (Eds.), *Science and pseudoscience in clinical psychology* (pp. 1–14). New York: Guilford Press.

Linehan, M. M. (1993). *Skills training manual for treating borderline personality disorder.* New York: Guilford Press.

Locke, E. A., & Latham, G. P. (1990). *A theory of goal setting and task performance.* Upper Saddle River, NJ: Prentice-Hall.

Lutkenhouse, J., Gardner, F. L., & Morrow, C. (2007). *A randomized controlled trial comparing the performance enhancement effects of Mindfulness-Acceptance-Commitment (MAC) performance enhancement and psychological skills training procedures.* Manuscript in preparation.

Lynch, T. R., Robins, C. J., Morse, J. Q., & MorKrause, E. D. (2001). A mediational model relating affect intensity, emotion inhibition, and psychological distress. *Behavior Therapy, 32,* 519–536.

Lyonfields, J. D., Borkovec, T. D., & Thayer, J. F. (1995). Vagal tone in generalized anxiety disorder and the effects of aversive imagery and worrisome thinking. *Behavior Therapy, 26,* 457–466.

Martens, R., Burton, D., Vealey, R. S., Bump, L. A., & Smith, D. E. (1990). Development and validation of the Competitive State Anxiety Inventory-2. In R. Martens, R. S. Vealey, & D. Burtons (Eds.), *Competitive anxiety in sport* (pp. 117–190). Champaign, IL: Human Kinetics.

Mayer, J. D., Salovey, P., & Caruso, D. (2004). Emotional intelligence: Theory, findings, and implications. *Psychological Inquiry, 15,* 197–215.

Maynard, I. W., Smith, M. J., & Warwick-Evans, L. (1995). The effects of a cognitive intervention strategy on competitive state anxiety and performance in semiprofessional soccer players. *Journal of Sport and Exercise Psychology, 17,* 428–446.

McNair, D., Lorr, M., & Dropplemen, L. (1971). *Profile of Mood States.* San Diego, CA: Educational and Industrial Testing Services.

McNally, I. M. (2002). Contrasting concepts of competitive state-anxiety in sport: Multidimensional anxiety and catastrophe theories. *Athletic Insight, 4.* Retrieved August 23, 2004, from http://www.athleticinsight.com/Vol4Iss2/Anxiety_Issue_2.htm

Meichenbaum, D. (1977). *Cognitive behaviour modification: An integrative approach.* New York: Plenum.

Mennin, S. D., Heimberg, R. G., Turk, C. L., & Fresco, D. H. (2005). Preliminary evidence for an emotion dysregulation model of generalized anxiety disorder. *Behaviour Research and Therapy, 43,* 1281–1310.

Meyer, T. J., Miller, M. L., Metzger, R. L., & Borkovec, T. D. (1990). Development and validation of the Penn State Worry Questionnaire. *Behaviour Research and Therapy, 28,* 487–495.

Meyers, A. W., Whelan, J. P., & Murphy, S. M. (1996). Cognitive behavioral strategies in athletic performance enhancement. In M. Hersen, R. M. Eisler, & P. M. Miller (Eds.), *Progress in behavior modification* (Vol. 30, pp. 137–164). Pacific Grove, CA: Brooks/Cole.

Miller, J. J., Fletcher, K., & Kabat-Zinn, J. (1995). Three-year follow-up and clinical implications of a mindfulness meditation-based stress reduction intervention in the treatment of anxiety disorders. *General Hospital Psychiatry, 17,* 192–200.

Moore, Z. E. (2003a). Ethical dilemmas in sport psychology: Discussion and recommendations for practice. *Professional Psychology: Research and Practice, 34,* 601–610.

Moore, Z. E. (2003b). Toward the development of an evidence based practice of sport psychology: A structured qualitative study of performance enhancement interventions (Doctoral dissertation, La Salle University, 2003). *Dissertation Abstracts International-B, 64,* 5227.

Murphy, S. M., & Wolfolk, R. (1987). The effects of cognitive interventions on competitive anxiety and performance on a fine motor skill accuracy task. *International Journal of Sport Psychology, 18,* 152–166.

Nideffer, R. M., & Sagal, M. (2001). *Assessment in sport psychology.* Morgantown, WV: Fitness Information Technology.

Novick-Kline, P., Turk, C. L., Mennin, S. D., Hoyt, E., & Gallagher, C. (2005). Level of emotional awareness as a differentiating variable between individuals with and without generalized anxiety disorder. *Journal of Anxiety Disorders, 19,* 557–572.

Orlick, T. (1989). Reflections on sportpsych consulting with individual and team sport athletes at summer and winter Olympic games. *The Sport Psychologist, 3,* 358–365.

Orlick, T., & Partington, J. (1988). Mental links to excellence. *The Sport Psychologist, 2,* 105–130.

Orsillo, S. M., & Roemer, E. (2005). *Acceptance and mindfulness-based approaches to anxiety: Conceptualization and treatment.* New York: Springer.

Perna, F., Neyer, M., Murphy, S. M., Ogilvie, B. C., & Murphy, A. (1995). Consultations with sport organizations: A cognitive-behavioral model. In S. M. Murphy (Ed.), *Sport psychology interventions* (pp. 235–252). Champaign, IL: Human Kinetics.

Prochaska, J. O., DiClemente, C. C., & Norcross, J. C. (1992). The transtheoretical approach. In J. C. Norcross & M. R. Goldfried (Eds.), *Handbook of psychotherapy integration* (pp. 300–334). New York: Basic Books.

Purdon, C. (1999). Thought suppression and psychopathology. *Behaviour Research and Therapy, 37,* 1029–1054.

Rapee, R. M. (1993). The utilization of working memory by worry. *Behaviour Research and Therapy, 31,* 617–620.

Rapee, R. M., & Lim, L. (1992). Discrepancy between self and observer ratings of performance in social phobics. *Journal of Abnormal Psychology, 101,* 728–731.

Ravizza, K. (1990). Sportpsych consultation issues in professional baseball. *The Sport Psychologist, 4,* 330–340.

Rich, A. R., & Woolever, D. K. (1988). Expectancy and self-focused attention: Experimental support for the self-regulation model of test anxiety. *Journal of Social and Clinical Psychology, 7,* 246–259.

Roemer, L., & Orsillo, S. M. (2002). Expanding our conceptualization of and treatment for general anxiety disorder: Integrating mindfulness/acceptance-based approaches with existing cognitive-behavioral models. *Clinical Psychology: Science and Practice, 9,* 27–44.

Rotella, R. J. (1990). Providing sport psychology consulting services to professional athletes. *The Sport Psychologist, 4,* 409–417.

Russell, W. D. (2001). An examination of flow state occurrence in college athletes. *Journal of Sport Behavior, 24,* 83–107.

Safran, J. D., & Segal, Z. V. (1990). *Interpersonal process in cognitive therapy.* Northvale, NJ: Jason Aronson.

Salazar, W., Landers, D. M., Petruzzello, S. J., & Han, M. (1990). Hemispheric asymmetry, cardiac response, and performance in elite archers. *Research Quarterly for Exercise and Sport, 61,* 351–359.

Sbrocco, T., & Barlow, D. H. (1996). Conceptualizing the cognitive component of sexual arousal: Implications for sexuality research and treatment. In P. M. Salkovskis (Ed.), *Frontiers of cognitive therapy* (pp. 419–449). New York: Guilford Press.

Segal, Z. V., Williams, J. M. G., & Teasdale, J. D. (2002). *Mindfulness-based cognitive therapy for depression.* New York: Guilford Press.

Smith, R. E. (1986). Toward a cognitive affective model of athletic burnout. *Journal of Sport Psychology, 8,* 36–50.

Smith, R. E. (1989). Applied sport psychology in an age of accountability. *Journal of Applied Sport Psychology, 1,* 166–180.

Smith, R. E., Smoll, F. L., & Schutz, R. W. (1990). Measurement and correlates of sport-specific cognitive and somatic trait anxiety: The Sport Anxiety Scale. *Anxiety Research, 2,* 263–280.

Spirito, A. (1999). Empirically supported treatments in pediatric psychology [Special issue]. *Journal of Pediatric Psychology, 24,* 87–174.

Stopa, L., & Clark, D. M. (1993). Cognitive processes in social phobia. *Behaviour Research and Therapy, 31,* 255–267.

Strean, W. B., & Roberts, G. C. (1992). Future directions in applied sport psychology research. *The Sport Psychologist, 6,* 55–65.

Swain, A. B. J., & Jones, G. (1996). Explaining performance variance: The relative contribution of intensity and direction dimensions of competitive state anxiety. *Anxiety, Stress, and Coping: An International Journal, 9,* 1–18.

Taylor, J., & Schneider, B. A. (1992). The Sport-Clinical Intake Protocol: A comprehensive interview instrument for applied sport psychology. *Professional Psychology: Research and Practice, 23,* 318–325.

Teachman, B. A., & Woody, S. R. (2004). Staying tuned to research in implicit cognition: Relevance for clinical practice with anxiety disorders. *Cognitive and Behavioral Practice, 11,* 149–159.

Teasdale, J. D., Segal, Z., & Williams, J. M. (1995). How does cognitive therapy prevent depressive relapse and why should attentional control (mindfulness) training help? *Behavior Research and Therapy, 33,* 25–39.

Turk, C. L., Heimberg, R. G., Lutarek, J. A., Mennin, D. S., & Fresco, D. M. (2005). Delineating emotion regulation deficits in generalized anxiety disorder: A comparison with social anxiety disorder. *Cognitive Therapy and Research, 29,* 89–106.

United States Olympic Committee Sport Psychology Staff. (1999). *Sport psychology mental training manual.* Colorado Springs: CO: USOC Sport Science and Technology Division.

Vealey, R. S. (1986). Conceptualization of sport confidence and competitive orientation: Preliminary investigation and instrument development. *Journal of Sport Psychology, 8,* 221–246.

Vealey, R. (1994). Current status and prominent issues in sport psychology interventions. *Medicine and Science in Sport and Exercise, 26,* 495–502.

Vealey, R. S., & Garner-Holman, M. (1998). Applied sport psychology: Measurement issues. In J. L. Duda (Ed.), *Advances in sport and exercise psychology measurements* (pp. 433–446). Morgantown, WV: Fitness Information Technology.

Wegner, D. M. (1994). Ironic processes of mental control. *Psychological Review, 101,* 34–52.

Weinberg, R. S. (2002). Goal setting in sport and exercise: Research to practice. In J. L. Van Raalte & B. W. Brewer (Eds.), *Exploring sport and exercise psychology* (2nd ed., pp. 25–48). Washington, DC: American Psychological Association.

Weinberg, R. S., Seabourne, T. G., & Jackson, A. (1981). Effects of visuo-motor behavior rehearsal, relaxation, and imagery on karate performance. *Journal of Sport Psychology, 3,* 228–238.

Wells, A. (2000). *Emotional disorders and metacognition: Innovative cognitive therapy.* New York: Wiley.

Whelan, J., Mahoney, M., & Meyers, A. (1991). Performance enhancement in sport: A cognitive-behavioral domain. *Behavior Therapy, 22,* 307–327.

Williams, J. M., & Leffingwell, T. R. (2002). Cognitive strategies in sport and exercise psychology. In J. L. Van Raalte & B. W. Brewer (Eds.), *Exploring sport and exercise psychology* (2nd ed., pp. 75–98). Washington, DC: American Psychological Association.

Wolanin, A. T. (2005). Mindfulness-Acceptance-Commitment (MAC) based performance enhancement for Division I collegiate athletes: A preliminary investigation (Doctoral dissertation, La Salle University, 2003). *Dissertation Abstracts International-B, 65,* pp. 3735–3794.

Woodman, T., & Hardy, L. (2001). Stress and anxiety. In R. N. Singer, H. A. Hausenblas, & C. M. Janelle (Eds.), *Handbook of sport psychology* (2nd ed., pp. 290–318). New York: Wiley.

Young, J. E. (1999). *Cognitive therapy for personality disorders: A schema-focused approach* (3rd ed.). Sarasota, FL: Professional Resource Press.

Young, J. E. (2002). The Young Schema Questionnaire: Short form. Retrieved January, 2006, from http://www.schematherapy.com

Young, J. E., Klosko, J. S., & Weishaar, M. E. (2003). *Schema therapy: A practitioner's guide.* New York: Guilford Press.

Zaichkowsky, L. D., & Baltzell, A. (2001). Arousal and performance. In R. N. Singer, H. A. Hausenblas, & C. M. Janelle (Eds.), *Handbook of sport psychology* (2nd ed., pp. 319–339). New York: Wiley.

Index

CPSIA information can be obtained at www.ICGtesting.com
Printed in the USA
BVOW06*0029160715

408816BV00002BA/3/P